If you've ever wondered about chiropractic and why it has become the number-one choice for drug-free, nonsurgical pain relief and improved physical performance, Dr. Ingham answers your questions. This insightful book dispels the myths and clarifies the science behind the chiropractic approach to health and wellness.

Mark Sanna, DC, ACRB Level II, FICC
President, Breakthrough Coaching

Dr. Ingham debunks the myths around chiropractic care by illustrating the education and science, while highlighting patient outcomes. This book, more than any other, gives the patient the information they need for a truly informed choice in natural health care for themselves and their families. This is the book that gets it right.

Dr. George Birnbach
Founder, Designed Clinical Nutrition

Thank you for this insightful book into the full benefits of chiropractic. I'm certain most have no idea regarding the facts you present here. Thank you for spreading the truth of alternate ways to health versus the standard drug therapy route.

Dr. Jay Morgan

Inspired by the treatment his mother received when he was growing up, Dr. Ingham tells his own personal story about how the chiropractic practices are effective and necessary in a world of "quick fixes" and overprescription of painkillers. Using very thorough research and Dr. Ingham's personal experiences, this book details how chiropractic medicine is a legitimate field that can treat patients more efficiently than traditional medicine.

Dr. Charles M. Rubert Pérez
Assistant Professor of Chemistry, DePaul University

T0098708

I have been actively training and competing in jiujitsu and sub-mission wrestling for over twenty years, and I have had my fair share of injuries that some would deem life altering or career ending, but fortunately enough, I am still actively training and competing thanks in large part to the chiropractic care of Dr. Ingham. Dr. Ingham has dedicated his life to healing and has been blessed with the hands of a healer. I am grateful to have been his patient for over ten years and am so excited that his message will reach more people through this book!

Adem Redzovic
Gracie Jiujitsu Black Belt

As a police officer, it's imperative to have a certain level of fitness. For me personally, the combination of strength training along with the physical tasks of being in law enforcement have led me to seek out proper maintenance for my body. Dr. Ingham's knowledge and adjustments have allowed me to weight train and be a productive police officer who feels great without pain. This book is a great read for any tactical athlete like myself!

David Regalado
Chicago Police Officer

The
TRUE
POWER
—— of ——
CHIROPRACTIC

*Unlock **Your Body's Natural Ability** to*
ADAPT, RENEW, *and* RESTORE

DR. JASON W. INGHAM, DC, CCSP

Published by Advantage, Charleston, South Carolina.
Member of Advantage Media Group.

ADVANTAGE is a registered trademark, and the Advantage colophon is a trademark of Advantage Media Group, Inc.

Printed in the United States of America.

10 9 8 7 6 5 4 3 2 1

ISBN: 978-1-64225-038-1
LCCN: 2019905305

Cover design by Melanie Cloth.
Layout design by Wesley Strickland.

This publication is designed to provide accurate and authoritative information in regard to the subject matter covered. It is sold with the understanding that the publisher is not engaged in rendering legal, accounting, or other professional services. If legal advice or other expert assistance is required, the services of a competent professional person should be sought.

 Advantage Media Group is proud to be a part of the Tree Neutral® program. Tree Neutral offsets the number of trees consumed in the production and printing of this book by taking proactive steps such as planting trees in direct proportion to the number of trees used to print books. To learn more about Tree Neutral, please visit www.treeneutral.com.

Advantage Media Group is a publisher of business, self-improvement, and professional development books and online learning. We help entrepreneurs, business leaders, and professionals share their Stories, Passion, and Knowledge to help others Learn & Grow. Do you have a manuscript or book idea that you would like us to consider for publishing? Please visit **advantagefamily.com** or call **1.866.775.1696**.

In loving memory of
Ruby Wanda Deel
"Nanny"

CONTENTS

INTRODUCTION

My mother was stunning. A woman with long, flowing blond hair, she was captivating enough to make anyone do a double take. Unfortunately, as apparent as her beauty was, so too were her physical limitations.

As an infant, Mom was diagnosed with polio. It was terrifying news at the time, considering that most infants who contracted the disease didn't survive. Mom, on the other hand, was a fighter. Her tiny body battled polio with the aid of doctors and medicine, but the disease didn't leave her unmarred. Instead, it left the right side of her body limp, weak, and defenseless.

At a young age, she spent several months living with the aid of an iron lung. Even after that time had passed and she began to flourish into an attractive young woman, the right side of her body served as a permanent reminder of the disease that had attempted to claim her life. The virus had multiplied in her nervous system, which prevented nerve cells from activating skeletal muscle, specifically in her right leg. This condition is termed *acute flaccid paralysis*. As a child, I remember the imbalance in her body. One leg was longer than the other because her hips were misaligned and her muscles were imbalanced. Seemingly simple tasks, like climbing the stairs, proved increasingly challenging with age. As she hobbled up, one step at a time, the pain and discomfort were evident in her delicate features.

Most kids my age were scolded or sent to their rooms as a form of punishment for bad behavior. My sister and I, however, were disciplined by being tasked with massaging Mom's aching muscles. Today, of course, I realize this was less of a penalty and more for her benefit as she tried to cope with musculoskeletal problems.

Despite her appreciation of these massages, Mom never pursued alternative medicines because Dad, a well-respected respiratory therapist in Michigan, didn't have faith in them. If there was one thing he had full faith in, it was traditional medicine and traditional medicine only. He pooh-poohed the thought of anything nontraditional and would shake his head in distaste.

My dad was my ultimate role model and one of the coolest guys I knew. He had a secretary and an office and our family had a nice, big house and seemingly plenty of money. Naturally, because I looked up to him, I absorbed his opinions and perspective on life, adopting many of his thoughts and insights as my own. His beliefs pertaining to medicine were one of them, prompting me to wrinkle my nose at the mention of nontraditional medicinal alternatives.

Dad's opinions influenced more than just my young mind; they also impacted the treatment Mom received. Because Dad was well connected in the medical community, Mom had the entire Bon Secours Hospital at her disposal, which, according to Dad, meant she was in the best medical hands possible.

From my perspective, however, her condition never improved. I still saw her struggle with the stairs, with walking, with lifting things. The pain on her face was as clear as day, triggering my own emotions and sympathy.

Dad's perspective, however, was distinguished from mine. In his eyes, Mom was under the best care—this was as good as it was ever going to get for her, and he was confident in that belief.

Little did he know he'd be proven wrong.

A LIFE-ALTERING, EYE-OPENING EXPERIENCE

When I was six, Mom and Dad divorced. With Dad no longer around to denigrate the idea, Mom started seeing a chiropractor, something my dad and several others in the medical profession considered "fake medicine" and ruled out as an insignificant, ineffective practice.

Initially, because I'd absorbed so many of my dad's beliefs, I recall having a negative outlook about her visit.

"We going to the snake charmer, Mom?" I'd often tease. However, because I knew it meant so much to her, I restrained the urge to voice my doubts about chiropractic.

During the sessions, I'd struggle to rein in my horror as the chiropractor, Dr. Semlow, grabbed hold of Mom's neck until the frightening sounds of clicks and pops resounded throughout the room. When he started treating her hips, we discovered some shocking news. Dr. Semlow shared that most people who have hip displacement have hips that are anywhere from zero to three millimeters misaligned. Mom, on the other hand, was a whopping thirty millimeters out of position—the most he'd ever seen.

To say it was scary to see her go through all this therapy would be an understatement, especially for someone like me who was already uneasy about it all from the start.

Regardless of my apprehension, Mom continued with her appointments, and soon I begrudgingly noticed a marked improvement in her movements. Diminished were the earlier, immediately visible signs of atrophy debilitating her body. The effects of the chiropractic treatment were apparent on more than just her physical progress. Mom's disposition changed. She appeared happier and more at ease than ever before.

Thinking back, I wonder how her life would have been different if she'd had chiropractic care from a young age—how high school would have played out for her, how prom might have been a different experience. Of one thing I'm sure: a good chiropractor would have transformed the course of her life.

Watching Mom undergo treatment after treatment taught me a great deal about the value and benefits of complementary and alternative medicine, so much so that it influenced my decision to pursue a career in chiropractic.

Alongside Mom's role in my decision, I won't deny that my dad also had a part to play. Growing up, I often sensed that he'd inhibited himself from pursuing a degree as a medical doctor because he had us to consider. I felt a part of him hoped he could live vicariously through me and have me fulfill the dream he'd left incomplete. Being in total awe of him, I was more than happy to study the medical field—just not in the way he'd hoped.

After my initial uneasiness and downright fear of chiropractic subsided, I loved the chiropractic environment much more than I did the sterile, tense, and formal hospital one I'd grown up in. In the hospital, I was constantly scolded, "Don't touch anything!" In Dr. Semlow's office I could jump around tables and be a kid. People were much happier in general in the chiropractic setting than they were at the hospital, and children were encouraged to touch things—like the spine model—and ask questions. Even the cuddly toys, like teddy bears, had vertebrae you could play with and explore.

Plus, I hated the stinging stench of antiseptic, bleach, and medical equipment that seemed permanently infused in the walls, floors, and surfaces of the hospital.

I remember myself taking in this vast difference and thinking, I want to be Dr. Semlow, enjoying happiness, health, and healing—not Dad or his buddies dealing with death and dying.

Many years later in 1997, when I announced that I'd been accepted into chiropractic school, Dad wasn't happy with my decision. Becoming a chiropractor, in his opinion, was like becoming a glorified massage therapist with several more years of school. He was hoping I'd be a brain surgeon.

Even today, while it's evident he's proud of me and all I've accomplished, he'll throw the occasional jab, saying, "What father doesn't want their son to be a brain surgeon?"

I've learned to deal with his disappointment because I've treated tens of thousands of patients firsthand and have seen how chiropractic care has transformed their lives. I've witnessed that it is indeed (contrary to some beliefs) a scientific approach. Patients have approached me with gratitude shining bright in their eyes to say, "I owe you my life," just because they're now able to enjoy simple pleasures most of us take for granted, like picking up their grandchildren, playing golf, or enjoying a good night's sleep.

AN EFFECTIVE APPROACH TO COMPLEMENTARY AND ALTERNATIVE MEDICINE

Back pain accounts for more than 264 million lost workdays in one year—that's two workdays for every full-time worker in the country.[1] When these workers trickle through the doors of medical offices, they leave no better than when they arrived—the only difference is they're

---

1   "The Hidden Impact of Musculoskeletal Disorders on Americans," US Bone and Joint Initiative, 2018.

"officially" diagnosed with lower back pain. However, this diagnosis doesn't identify the cause of the pain. It doesn't tell you why the pain exists—just that it's there.

Often traditional doctors may suggest painkillers to numb the nervous system so patients can get through the day. They're hoping the problem will resolve itself, which it typically doesn't. The pain does generally subside, but the problem remains until it is ignored for so long that surgery is their last option.

Many medical practitioners I know practice what I call the "hope and poke" approach. They admit to being unaware of how to effectively treat back pain so, through their own admissions, they throw medication at it. If that doesn't work, they prescribe physical therapy. As a last resort, they send patients to a pain specialist.

Chiropractors, on the other hand, work to identify why the back pain exists and how it can effectively be treated. They have profound knowledge about how the spinal column is connected to the entire body and understand just how vital alignment is for the body to function optimally. The knowledge these professionals wield can not only have a profound impact on patients but it can also transform how health care is administered in the US. We'll talk more about that in chapter 1.

All I ask for now is that you keep an open mind. I've had people come to me and say, "I don't know if I believe in chiropractic."

My response to them is always the same: "That's okay. You don't have to believe. It's not a religion, so it'll still work on you, even if you don't have faith in it."

I've found that once they get the care they need, they become believers.

WHY BELIEVE A WORD I SAY?

If you're asking this question, you're on the right track. To trust me, you should know more about me.

I started practicing chiropractic in 2000, but my story actually started a little before that in 1995, when I graduated with degrees in psychology, biology, and anatomy from Wayne State University. Wayne State is an allied health school, which means it concentrates on medical areas of study with a robust premedical curriculum. Much of the undergraduate student population continues to grad school to become doctors, nurses, pharmacists, and dentists. Even then, it had little information about chiropractic—not a single book in its massive library.

However, I wasn't going to let that deter me. Instead, I started getting creative in my approach to gain the information and knowledge I craved. I began hunting out chiropractic physicians, making appointments with them, and offering to take them out to lunch so that I could get inside their heads and learn more about the fascinating field of chiropractic.

Perhaps the greatest resource I had was Dr. Semlow himself. He's the one who instructed me on where to find books and resources that piqued my interest.

Finally, in 1999, I earned a doctoral degree from Parker University in Dallas, Texas. I continued studying while in private practice, earning my postdoctoral distinction in sports medicine in 2003 from the National University of Health Sciences. My first position as a chiropractic physician was practicing in a place I hoped never to work—an antiseptic- and bleach-swathed hospital. At the time, the medical industry hadn't quite figured out how doctors and chiropractic could collaborate, or where complementary and alternative medicine even fit into the bigger picture. Today, it's only a slightly different story.

One of the requirements for my doctoral degree was to generate thirty new patients in a single year, a challenge I embraced whole-heartedly in hopes of soon launching my own practice. My strategy was simple but proved extremely effective.

I was a group instructor at a local fitness studio, so I got several chiropractic T-shirts and started wearing them during my instruction sessions—a subtle tactic, but it worked. Suddenly, people at the gym started getting curious about chiropractic care and began asking me questions. I'd explain to them how it worked and encourage them to sign up for a consultation. Eventually, many of them would become new patients.

As a result of my strategy, I was one of the first in my class to fulfill the requirement—and within only three months. My speedy success got my mind churning: if I could generate this many new patients simply by wearing T-shirts while teaching spin classes or aerobics, imagine what I could do if I opened a clinic right inside the gym.

With this idea brewing in my mind, I quit the hospital after only a year, got a loan from my mom, and opened Advanced Spine & Sports Care in an eight-hundred-square-foot facility inside a Bally Total Fitness Club in 2001.

It was fantastic. And business was brisk.

I was working with athletes I had trained the previous three years while in school, and I couldn't think of a better place to be.

However, soon I stumbled into a minor, but pleasant, problem: my practice was outgrowing the facility. I acted quickly, opening another practice in uptown Chicago, but soon realized that managing two practices wasn't the life I wanted.

Suddenly, I'd transformed from Dr. Ingham to Employee Manager Ingham—and managing in itself is a whole field of study that takes years to master and took me away from the patient care I loved, so managing two locations was a challenge I wasn't up for.

Lucky for me, the problem ended up resolving itself. A few years in, the Bally Total Fitness Corporation folded, taking my clinic with it, so I doubled the size of my uptown Chicago practice to 3,200 square feet.

Today, my office is staffed with one part-time and two full-time chiropractors, an athletic trainer, a rehab specialist, and several chiropractic assistants—all of whom I consider my family.

My vision for the practice is clear: to serve people and help them live a better, pain-free, and painkiller-free life.

As you can see, I have years of experience and an immense interest in the field. I've treated thousands of patients, and my hope is to help you understand that there's a world of complementary and alternative medicine out there that can change the way you live.

This book is a straightforward, no-holds-barred account and a compilation of valuable data. I hope that by reading it, you'll start thinking differently about how to take care of yourself and the ones you love, and that you will understand that you have more options than you think. I hope you'll get upset and ask questions. And when things look bleak and you're contemplating reaching for that pill because you need an increased dose of pain medicine, I hope you'll understand that there is a better way.

Chapter 1

TODAY'S HEALTH CARE CRISIS

According to the National Institute on Drug Abuse, 115
Americans die every day from opioid overdoses.[2]
From July 2016 through September 2017, opioid overdoses
increased 30 percent in forty-five states, according to the Centers
for Disease Control and Prevention (CDC). In the Midwest
alone, they spiked 70 percent during that same period.[3]

Government leaders talk about jailing or executing drug dealers as solutions to opioid abuse, but contrary to popular belief, the spate of opioid addiction doesn't come from seedy dealers operating in dark alleys. Many times, it's the result of how our current health care system approaches pain management.

---

2   "Overdose deaths involving opioids, by type of opioid, United States, 2000–2016," Centers for Disease Control and Prevention/National Center for Health Statistics, 2017.

3   "Opioid overdoses treated in emergency departments," Centers for Disease Control and Prevention, https://www.cdc.gov/vitalsigns/opioid-overdoses/index.html.

GAPS IN THE HEALTH CARE ARENA

Today's medical system is set up around the path of least resistance, encouraging patients to choose the easiest, most affordable options. Health insurance covers a large percentage of the cost for a doctor's visit and much of the cost of prescription drugs. However, it covers very little for physical therapy, and even less—if anything—for alternative/natural health care.

Add to that the fact that the musculoskeletal system is not taught particularly well in medical school, and you'll understand why so many medical doctors don't know how to deal with problems related to physical medicine. Often, these professionals will see only one chapter in a textbook about physical medicine and rehab, learning very little about complementary and alternative treatment possibilities.

In fact, a recent survey of 104 US medical schools backs this claim, proving the limited exposure medical students receive to this field:

- Approximately 20 percent offered no pain education.

- Only four schools, or 3.8 percent, had a required course on pain.

- Forty-four of the schools, or 42 percent, covered pharmacological pain management.

- The average number of hours devoted to pharmacological pain management, if any, was 0.7 hours.

- Only 35 percent of the schools addressed nonpharmacological pain management, including counseling, conservative pain treatments, evidence-based complementary and alternative medicine, and rehabilitation of pain.

- The average number of hours devoted to nonpharmacological pain management was a mere 1.1.[4]

Another study found that 82 percent of incoming interns at the University of Pennsylvania failed a test about musculoskeletal disorders because they didn't have enough knowledge to accurately diagnose and/or treat such disorders.[5]

As you can see, these numbers don't work in our favor when it comes to helping patients treat pain.

THE AVERAGE JOE'S APPROACH TO PAIN TREATMENT

Because of the limited education they receive about the musculoskeletal system, most physicians admit to not being adequately prepared to treat chronic pain. Of five hundred primary care physicians surveyed in a different study, only 34 percent felt comfortable treating musculoskeletal problems—and the competence of even those 34 percent was questionable. In fact, one study found no relationship between physicians' self-assessments of their knowledge against their ability to treat pain and the quality of their treatment decisions.[6]

---

4   L. Mezei, B. Murinson, and Johns Hopkins Pain Curriculum Development Team, "Pain education in North American schools," *Journal of Pain* 12, no. 12 (2011): 1199–1208.

5   Nathan W. Skelley et al., "Medical student musculoskeletal education: An institutional survey," *Journal of Bone and Joint Surgery* 94, no. 19:e146 (2012): 1–7.

6   J. E. O'Rorke et al., "Physicians' comfort in caring for patients with chronic nonmalignant pain," *American Journal of Medical Sciences* 333, no. 2 (2007): 93–100.

As a result of their limited knowledge, most medical doctors offer a diagnosis of lower back pain when they encounter a suffering patient, when the pain itself doesn't help to identify the cause of the concern. They advise patients that the pain will subside with time if left alone or, worse, they tell them it's in their heads. Often, they'll tell the patient that back pain is a normal part of getting older.

Cavities are normal too, but no one wants one. A cavity hurts like hell if left untreated. So does back pain. And your back is involved in far more of your overall wellness than a tooth.

To numb the back pain until it hopefully "disappears," doctors prescribe painkillers. However, the pain is not caused by a lack of an opioid or medication in your body; it is the result of a problem. Patients come to me all the time, saying, "The doctor didn't even listen to me; he just pulled out a prescription pad." This take on pain management is what I call the "hope and poke" approach—simply turning off the problem at the central nervous system level to dull the system against pain.

The process starts with over-the-counter pills that doctors often throw at the problem to see what happens. However, according to studies, these don't offer much relief:

Painkillers such as aspirin, Aleve, and Advil don't help most people with back pain, a new review finds. The researchers estimated that only one in six people gained a benefit from taking these nonsteroidal anti-inflammatory drugs (NSAIDs). Meanwhile, previous research has suggested that another common painkiller, Tylenol (acetaminophen), isn't very useful either, the study authors added. The findings raise the prospect that no over-the-counter painkillers really ease back pain, at least in the short term, and some may raise the risk of gastrointestinal problems. "There are other effective and safer strategies to manage spinal pain," said review author Gustavo Machado.[7]

This "solution" of tossing drugs at the pain is nothing more than a way to sidestep the true cause of the problem. Perhaps worse than that, this approach can take you down a treacherous path.

A PROBLEM THAT CAN SPIRAL BEYOND JUST PAIN

In most cases where doctors prescribe drugs, patients return at a later date, reporting no improvements in condition. Again, instead of uncovering the underlying problem, the doctor masks the pain, this time with a stronger dosage of medication. Finally, the patient experiences a decrease in pain, because the opioid is dulling their nervous system. However, the problem is that it's targeting not only their back but their nervous system as a whole, so that if they were punched in the face, they wouldn't feel that either.

This approach has very real dangers for a simple reason: the higher dosage becomes ineffective over time. The body's tolerance to the drug increases, and soon the pain is back and you find yourself headed to the doctor … again.

At that point, your doctor likely ups the dosage even more—to a certain point. Remember, from the doctor's perspective, pain is just a normal part of life, or it's in your head.

---

7   "Common painkillers don't ease back pain, study finds," HealthDay, last updated February 2, 2017, https://consumer.healthday.com/bone-and-joint-information-4/backache-news-53/common-painkillers-don-t-ease-back-pain-study-finds-719292.html.

Eventually, they might realize that you feel the need for an increased dosage because you're abusing the drug—opioids are extremely easy to get hooked on. By the time the realization strikes, they may be right. According to a study in the medical journal *Pain*, 21 to 29 percent of patients prescribed opioids for chronic pain misuse them.[8]

However, that's not the end of the story. Most patients grow desperate, sometimes turning to a buddy to see if they have leftover Oxycontin from a previous procedure, or visiting a different doctor to complain of the pain. More than half (53 percent) of prescription opioid users admit to getting their last painkillers from a friend or relative, with 40.4 percent paying nothing for the pills, according to the Center for Behavioral Health Statistics and Quality (CBHSQ).[9]

One step leads to another, and before we know, there are housewives in Plano, Texas, cooking up this crap (in the form of fentanyl) in their kitchens.

The results? Drug overdoses from overly powerful or incorrectly formulated opioids or progression to heroin. Eighty percent of people who use heroin first misused prescription drugs, according to the CBHSQ.[10] And one in five people know someone who's died

---

8   K. E. Vowles et al., "Rates of opioid misuse, abuse, and addiction in chronic pain: a systematic review and data synthesis," *Pain* 156, no. 4 (April 2015): 579–76, https://doi.org/. https://www.ncbi.nlm.nih.gov/pubmed/25785523.

9   "Key substance use and mental health indicators in the United States: results from the 2016 National Survey on Drug Use and Health," Substance Abuse and Mental Health Services Administration, September 2017, https://www.samhsa.gov/data/sites/default/files/NSDUH-FFR1-2016/NSDUH-FFR1-2016.pdf.

10   P. K. Muhuri, J. C. Gfroerer, and M. C. Davies, "Associations of nonmedical pain reliever use and initiation of heroin use in the United States," CBHSQ Data Review, August 2013, https://www.samhsa.gov/data/sites/default/files/DR006/DR006/nonmedical-pain-reliever-use-2013.htm.

from an opioid overdose.[11]

However, the people dealing with this problem aren't just numbers or statistics to me—and probably not to you either.

THE SAD REALITY BEHIND THE VICIOUS CYCLE

When I was about five years into practice, a professional ballet dancer came in for treatment with her family. She had been hard on her feet and body, as most athletes are, and she was taking a lot of painkillers to mask the pain. Some days she would come in with her mouth so dry from the painkillers that she couldn't even speak, and some days she was nearly incapacitated.

I was still young and meek and I didn't really know how to get her help for her opioid problem. For that matter, I wasn't even sure if she really even had a problem. It was a dirty, unspoken secret and a crazy, terrible situation for her to be in. I didn't try hard enough to convince her that she was taking the wrong approach to deal with her pain.

Then one day, I attended her funeral—she had overdosed. This still bothers me. I felt like I could have done better. I could have taught her more about the hazards of the opioids she was relying on.

Now, I'm very outspoken about the dangers of opioid use—and the more favorable alternatives.

Unfortunately, in the medical community at large, little is being done about the opioid crisis, even though experts acknowledge the

---

11 "1 in 5 Americans Say They Know Someone Who Has Died from Prescription Painkiller Overdose," Kaiser Family Foundation, accessed January 18, 2018, https://www.kff.org/other/slide/1-in-5-americans-say-they-know-someone-who-has-died-from-prescription-painkiller-overdose.

problem exists. For instance, major medical organizations have suggested new standards and different approaches to pain assessment and management, particularly when it comes to the use of drugs. In 2011, the Institute of Medicine issued a position statement that talked about imperatives for early integration of nonpharmacological approaches by practitioners for the treatment of pain—in other words, recommending a non-drug-based approach to pain.[12]

Later, in 2014, the Academic Consortium for Complementary and Alternative Health Care issued a statement in support of non-pharmacological strategies as a way to reduce opioid use.[13]

An article in the *Journal of General Internal Medicine* lists spinal manipulation as one of nine non–drug therapies to be used first for chronic pain.[14]

An article in the *Family Practice Journal* recommended patients seek chiropractic care for musculoskeletal lower back pain before turning to traditional medical care.[15]

The medical community is starting to recognize the problem. Awareness is driven by the heroin and fentanyl overdoses that are killing people at a higher rate than ever before.

---

12 Institute of Medicine, *Relieving Pain in America: A Blueprint for Transforming Prevention, Care, Education, and Research* (Washington, DC: National Academies Press, 2011).

13 M. Menard et al., "Never Only Opioids," PAINS Project, September 24, 2014.

14 B. Kligler et al., "Clinical policy recommendations from the VHA state-of-the-art conference on non-pharmacological approaches to chronic musculoskeletal pain," *Journal of General Internal Medicine* 33, Suppl 1 (2018): 16. https://doi.org/10.1007/s11606-018-4323-z.

15 "Nonpharmacologic treatment of chronic pain: What works?" *The Journal of Family Practice*. 67, no. 8 (August 2018): 474–477, 480–483.

However, change is a slow process. And if someone isn't regularly restating or reinforcing these alternative-treatment-first statements, they'll mean very little.

It goes back to educating the physician, educating the consumer, and being able to access these nonpharmacological approaches. However, frontline medical providers often don't know enough about the musculoskeletal system and treatment options to point you in the right direction, or they're dismissive of what they consider "lesser treatments." (We'll talk about that more in chapter 2.)

Unfortunately, the current system, by default, delivers you the pharmacological answer, and that's a bad start.

Failure to disclose risks and dangers of dangerous medications is commonplace, even in published research conducted for large manufacturers by well-educated medical researchers. In fact, GlaxoSmith-Kline, Eli Lilly, and Johnson & Johnson have all been fined by the Food and Drug Administration for such omissions.

Of course, there's also another problem: big pharma is powerful, and its marketing initiatives are educating consumers far more effectively than physicians are.

PHARMACEUTICAL INDUSTRIES: THE BIG KAHUNAS BEHIND THE DRUG PROBLEM

Companies in the pharma industry spend a lot of money and time enticing doctors with gifts so that they'll prescribe their drugs. They also expend endless dollars trying to persuade patients that they need these drugs. Once these patients buy into the propaganda and are convinced these medications are exactly what they need, they insist on the prescription, visiting different doctors until they find one who's willing to prescribe it. As an aside, the money these companies spend on marketing must be recouped through increased drug costs, which adds to the difficulty of decreasing health care costs.

From a chiropractic perspective, we've known from the get-go that this is all a recipe for disaster.

Don't get me wrong: prescription drugs have made remarkable impacts. Just look at how far we have come with HIV. This diagnosis is no longer a death sentence but rather a manageable condition with the use of the proper medications and medical management. While there are certainly many areas for medicine to leave its mark, the musculoskeletal arena isn't one of them.

Are there other steps, beyond numbing, that traditional medicine takes to combat musculoskeletal pain? Yes, but they're not necessarily better or more effective.

If a patient still has pain after six weeks of treatment with medication, the doctor might recommend physical therapy—although, again, with no diagnosis whatsoever. Maybe the doctor will give the physical therapist a semblance of structure or plan for the treatment, but often that doesn't happen, leaving the therapist to guess at what they are treating and risk missing the mark completely.

How exactly does this happen? If the primary care doctor isn't fully confident in their knowledge of the musculoskeletal system (we'll get into this shortly), they can't provide a proper diagnosis or even a bigger picture of what is going on in order to help guide the physical therapist with the treatment plan.

Whenever a doctor orders physical therapy treatment, or anything for that matter, they must provide what is called an ICD-10 code. This code is used not only for insurance purposes, but it states the doctor's diagnosis. This diagnosis is then available to the physical therapist. If the primary care doctor understands the true cause of a patient's pain and the diagnosis is accurate, the physical therapy treatment can be spot on.

However, if the diagnosis isn't accurate, this puts the physical therapist in a tough position. They must treat based on the doctor's diagnosis, but the physical therapist, who is trained to treat musculoskeletal disorders, may realize the problem is actually something else entirely. As I write this book, physical therapists do not have the legal ability to diagnose problems or disorders, although physical therapy associations are fighting for this change. Currently, if the initial diagnosis by the primary care doctor is wrong, it's only hurting the patient involved. This approach has proven to lead to less-than-great outcomes, as numerous statistics have shown.

SURGERY: AS GOOD AS GAMBLING

Then there's surgery. Each year, the existence of unnecessary surgery remains a daunting reality that continues to expose our patients to unjustified surgical risk, not to mention possible complications and downtime with minimal gain.[16] Multiple clinical trials have shown that spinal fusions for back pain do not lead to improved long-term patient outcomes when compared to nonoperative treatment modalities.[17, 18]

---

16   Gina Kolata, "Why 'useless surgery' is still popular," *New York Times*, August 3, 2016.

17   A. Raabe, J. Beck, and C. Ulrich, "Necessary or unnecessary? A critical glance on spine surgery" [German], *Therapeutische Umschau* 71 (2014): 701–705, https://doi.org/10.1024/0040-5930/a000614.

18   S. V. Srinivas, R. A. Deyo, and Z. D. Berger, "Application of 'less is more' to low back pain," *Archives of Internal Medicine* 172 (2012): 1016–1020, https://doi.org/10.1001/archinternmed.2012.1838.

When you go through invasive surgery, there's really no way to know whether you'll get better. It's a coin toss. Yet, people spend hundreds of thousands of dollars on surgeries to this day.

This begs the question: Why do we continue to do unnecessary surgeries, most of which have chances of success no better than a coin toss, not to mention deal with the significant downtime, serious risks, and possible complications that accompany them? Because that is what surgeons have been trained to do, what they've always done; they simply don't know of a better way. Or, more discouragingly, because they're incentivized to perform surgical procedures for financial gain, renown, or both.[19]

Study upon study shows how ineffective surgery is, how ineffective opioids are, and how ineffective medical treatment, in general, is for musculoskeletal problems. Doing what we're doing because that's what we've always done is no longer the answer.

In fact, medical treatment as currently practiced can be detrimental to your overall health. According to the CDC, the three leading causes of death in the United States are the following:[20]

- Heart disease (about 635,260 deaths per year)

- Cancer (about 598,038 deaths per year)

- Medical errors (about 161,374 deaths per year)

When medical errors top the list as the third leading cause, something's wrong. Not only are these errors avoidable, but their very existence also has a detrimental impact on the cost of health care. Because of medical errors, physicians and specialists have to pay exorbitant amounts on malpractice insurance. The premiums for the

---

19 P. F. Stahel, *Blood, Sweat and Tears—Becoming a Better Surgeon* (Shropshire, England: TFM Publishing, 2016) 320.

20 *Journal of Patient Safety* 9 (2013): 122–8.

policy are based on previous usage of the insurance and work a lot like home insurance.

Say, for instance, your home insurance is tied to your address—your premium could spike if the previous owner had a plumbing issue and filed a homeowner's claim before you even put an offer on the house.

It's the same for physicians; their usage of the malpractice policy determines their premiums for the following year, and those costs aren't cheap. Malpractice can vary by specialty, location, and the number of claims made. For each specialty, the actuaries also consider the severity of the claims and the cost to defend. A doctor of internal medicine in Cook County, Illinois, can pay as much as $40,000 a year; a general surgeon can pay as much as $120,000 a year; and an OB-GYN can pay as much as $177,000 per year.[21]

Physicians have little choice but to pass these costs on to you, the consumer. Just like with pharmaceutical marketing costs.

LIVING IN TIMES WHEN INSURANCE PROVIDES NO ASSURANCE

Compared to other first-world countries, our health care system is designed for people who have money—or really good insurance. The cost of treatment for patients with low back pain in the United States is estimated to be $240 billion per year.[22] With the rising cost of health care, the percentage you pay is rising even more quickly.

---

21 "Medical malpractice insurance by specialty: costs, statistics, and notable facts," accessed October 21, 2018, https://www.capson.com/medical-malpractice-insurance-by-specialty/.

22 E. Yelin, "Cost of musculoskeletal diseases: impact of work disability and functional decline" [review]. *Journal of Rheumatology Supplement* 68 (2003): 8–11.

Suddenly a $500 deductible, which used to be common, is now considered a godsend.

You're probably familiar with how much your employer deducts from your paycheck, or how much you pay out of pocket for insurance premiums each month, and you probably also know that this amount is only increasing. Year after year the amount of money you're spending at the doctor's office is also going up, because of copays, coinsurance, and deductibles—and you're getting less for paying more.

I don't know anyone who says they're getting their money's worth from their insurance—not even the people who used to think they had good insurance.

At one point, patients would come to my office confident that their insurance would cover everything. When someone says that today, my first reaction is to check with their insurance company, because I know that's not the case. No copay? No deductible? No way. Those days are long gone.

It's funny: BlueCross BlueShield still makes these commercials with smiling patients talking about how the insurance covers their medical needs. Taking it a step further, they present happy doctors using taglines such as, "When you're covered by BlueCross BlueShield, you're family." It's laughable. It may give you the warm and fuzzies inside, but it's not even close to the truth.

Today, I could compare BlueCross BlueShield to a modern-day Mercedes. Back in the day, a Mercedes was an expensive car owned by only wealthy people. Now they have an entry-level Mercedes that is the same price as an entry-level Ford. It's an underpowered car, and it's nothing like what you'd get if you were to spend the kind of money that Mercedes is really known for, but it has the Mercedes logo on it.

It's the same concept with BlueCross BlueShield. Sure, it has great benefits packages, but it also has policies that have a $10,000 deductible and 70 percent coinsurance. Which policy you have is determined by how much money you, or your employer, can dedicate to the premium.

Now even preferred provider organization (PPO) plans, which used to allow you the flexibility of going anywhere you wanted for treatment, are like health maintenance organization (HMO) plans. Traditionally, if you had a Preferred Provider Organization (PPO) plan, you were able to see any type of doctor you wanted, such as a specialist, without having a referral from your primary care doctor. You could even see doctors outside of your network and insurance may still cover it. As a result, PPO plans usually have higher premiums and deductibles, but much more flexibility.

HMO plans, on the other hand, prevent you from seeing a specialist without first seeing your PCP and having a referral. If you see another doctor outside of your network, insurance won't cover it. While an HMO plan is more rigid, it typically has lower premiums and deductibles as a result.

It's not so much the case anymore. If you have a PPO plan now, you might still be subjected to preauthorization, and you might find your network getting smaller and smaller. In short, you're paying a PPO price but getting an HMO policy, plus there's the possibility of the insurance denying you services because they're not "medically necessary." Medical utilization review companies such as OrthoNet and American Specialty Health Network, just to name a few, try to cut costs by creating additional hoops for patients and providers to jump through before they cover services.

For example, a patient may pay for an insurance plan that covers twenty visits of chiropractic services, but after the twelfth visit, the patient and their provider are required to produce the notes and claims for medical necessity. This is a stall tactic and a way to deny services until someone complains and makes a stink, making it harder and more costly for patients to receive care.

At a time when health care costs are spiraling out of control, your insurance isn't really paying for your medical needs. Today, having an insurance card means virtually nothing.

However, the problems related to health care venture far beyond costs, stemming from the way medicine is practiced in the office.

GETTING TO THE ROOT OF THE ISSUE

One of the most common things new patients say to me after they seek a traditional medical solution is "I'm not being heard. No one's listening to what I'm saying." And they're right. Modern medicine is about getting people in and out to meet patient quotas, pumping up the bottom line, or simply covering the cost of practicing. The lack of reimbursement leads to needing to see X number of patients per hour. As a result, doctors can spend only a minuscule amount of time listening to each patient's needs.

I understand that health care is a business, but we're forgetting that these are people we're caring for—someone's mother, sister, brother, or loved one.

Conversely, although giving a chiropractic adjustment takes about two minutes, my sessions are a minimum of thirty minutes of face-to-face time with a dedicated member of my staff. The consultation part of the appointment should take, in my opinion, longer than any other part of the treatment. What a patient tells me is so much more valuable than any orthopedic test or exam I can perform.

Additionally, I make myself available through email for patients to reach out about their conditions or any questions they may have. They are not routed through a nurse case manager who may or may not understand their needs.

However, the modern doctor's office doesn't allow for that kind of interaction. As a result, patients feel like they're not being listened to. They feel like they're not valued. They feel as though the doctor is too busy and very unavailable.

The same impersonal care extends to lab tests, which are usually interpreted by computers. If the results are within a range that wouldn't necessarily be accurate to your specific person—a range written in some textbook somewhere—the doctor won't be alerted to a problem. Since those numbers aren't specific to you, it's easy for computers to miss something significant.

I can't even count the number of times I've caught things that computers have overlooked. In worst-case scenarios, this oversight has led to patients being put on conflicting medications because they're going to different physicians who aren't talking to each other.

This "get-them-in-get-them-out" mentality has led to medical care becoming a commodity, causing patients to price shop for the cheapest service. Most people decide that if they're going to get a prescription, they want to do it the easiest, most affordable way—by being able to call in their prescriptions, preferably without seeing a doctor.

Granted, there are situations when that may be appropriate. However, in my opinion, eight out of ten times it's not. Health care shouldn't be just about refilling medication. Health care should be about creating a relationship with someone who understands what's going on and who knows what you need before you need it. Counseling a patient on how to discontinue the use of medications should be the rule, not the exception. Yet, the message patients most often walk away with is "Here's your high cholesterol medication—enjoy that meal at McDonald's!"

I have a personal example of that shortcoming. One day Mom got sick and was being treated in a hospital. She had a primary care physician, but she needed additional physicians within the hospital that specialized in different disciplines and could assist in her care. We soon found out that the various specialties were not only not communicating with each other, but it was also evident that they didn't personally take the time to even review her chart or medical history. Mom was supposed to be taken care of, but instead, this added to both her stress and mine. It left me feeling very frustrated with the medical community. This is how we treat the sick?

Your personal health care doesn't have to be this way. You have more options than you might realize, and taking advantage of those options—such as seeing a chiropractor before you go for pain pills or surgery—can benefit you, without precluding you from trying more traditional medical approaches if need be.

I'm not saying I can fix every one of the people I see, but you owe it to yourself to determine whether there's a natural solution before wading into the insurance bureaucracy, taking pills, or getting invasive surgery. I get it; you're in pain. Of course, I want to help relieve your pain, but more importantly, I want to correct the problem, and if I can't fix it, I want to help you find someone who can. That's what a "doctor" is to me! I can become an advocate for you and make sure that we quickly find someone who can help.

You must try chiropractic first. Create a team of health care practitioners and make that the rule rather than the exception.

Don't be like the thirty-year-old professional soccer player who came to see me. This man had injured his back while playing and had a bulging disc, which is one of the most common problems chiropractic can solve. Unfortunately, his insurance didn't cover my services—but it did cover a surgery, so he went that route. Although I didn't agree with his decision and voiced my concerns, I understood he had to do what he had to do.

Eight months later, I walked into the exam room and there he was—bawling. The surgery hadn't helped at all. In fact, the pain was worse. He couldn't play soccer anymore, and his wife had left him. (I'm not sure how or if those events were connected, but nonetheless.)

"I'll pay double, triple," he begged. "Take care of me. Help me. Do anything you can."

At that point, he had hardware installed in his back, including four screws. There was nothing I could do.

If he'd only chosen to seek chiropractic first, I'm confident I could have helped him avoid surgery and get back on that soccer field.

If he'd given me thirty days to take care of him, this story might have had a happier ending. Thirty days. It's not crazy. It's not long. But it can make all the difference.

CHAPTER TAKEAWAYS:

- The modern approach to medical care is creating a health care crisis in this country: addiction to prescription drugs, unnecessary and ineffective surgery, and high cost of treatment.

- Your insurance is covering less for your treatment and medication than ever before, leaving you with more out-of-pocket expenses. Choose where to spend your money wisely.

- The current medical model has made health care treatments a commodity, and doctors don't have time to sit and listen to their patients.

- There is a better way. Try chiropractic first! Create a health care team!

Chapter 2

REAL DOCTOR?
SO MUCH MORE

As you'll recall from the intro, when I told my father I was going into chiropractic, he disparagingly commented that I was setting out to become a "glorified massage therapist."

"Why don't you want me to become a chiropractor?" I'd ask.

His response: "I don't know. I heard (blah, blah, blah)."

I quit listening after "I heard." It was apparent to me that he felt the way he did because he was uneducated about chiropractic. He'd heard things that may or may not have been accurate, perhaps even based on someone else's speculation or interpretation of what happens in a chiropractor's office.

Dad is far from the only person who doesn't understand what a chiropractor is and has a misguided perception of what we do. For instance, I can't tell you how many times I've heard that chiropractors aren't "real doctors."

What does that even mean? What is a real doctor? Does the authority to prescribe medicine make someone a "real doctor"? Or the ability to perform surgeries?

I'll grant that chiropractors aren't in traditional health care, but we're not exactly alternative health either. We're in this gray area that's a blend of the two.

When I hear the "not a real doctor" remark, I want to laugh. Sure, I'm not a medical doctor—that's true; my title is doctor of chiropractic. I don't prescribe drugs, and I don't do surgeries.

However, when it comes to neurology, alignment, and musculoskeletal disorders (injuries and disorders that affect the body's movement or musculoskeletal system, such as spinal disc disorders, carpal tunnel syndrome, ligament sprains, and tension neck syndrome), doctors of chiropractic are more thoroughly trained than any of those other "real doctors." In other words, we're spinal engineers. We spend years learning about one thing and one thing only—musculoskeletal pain and dysfunction—making us the ideal portal-of-entry provider for musculoskeletal disorders.

Ask me to identify a heart murmur and I would tell you that skill takes years to develop. What I am confident in is my ability to determine a normal heart rhythm from an abnormal one and refer you to someone who deals with heart disorders every day—a cardiologist. I don't treat medical conditions. I allow your body to heal itself and align it so that it can function optimally. Once, during a consultation to a nephrology fellow, I was explaining the anatomy of her spine and respectfully said, "I'm sure you know all this already."

She replied, "I'm a kidney specialist; I don't know anything about the spine."

"Great," I replied, "I'm a spine specialist. I don't know much about the kidneys."

CHIROPRACTORS ARE DOCTORS TOO

I frequently speak in front of crowds at meetings and conventions. Often, afterward, someone will approach me and say, "You're a chiropractor? Wow. You seem so knowledgeable." I wonder why that surprises them. Chiropractic isn't a weekend course; it's not some online certification.

Going through traditional medical school and chiropractic school is very similar, with the primary difference being that medical students complete residency programs and chiropractors enter internship programs. Postdoctoral degree specializations are offered in both disciplines.

The premedical prerequisites to get into chiropractic school are the same as medical school, meaning you have to enroll in a year of biology, a year of chemistry, a year of physics, a year of calculus, a year of organic chemistry, and a year of labs. As a result, most chiropractors have a four-year undergraduate degree in a science field.

While getting into chiropractic school tends to be less difficult, staying in is grueling. Chiropractic school has a high attrition rate. Consider this: 130 students entered Parker University with me; only about 100 graduated. Some fell behind, and others completely dropped out.

When I was in chiropractic school, the first two years were classroom study. The third year was a mixture of classroom and clinical, and the last year was all clinical. That first year, which consisted of all basic sciences, was the hardest of my life. I was in school from 7 a.m. to 5 p.m. Monday through Friday, and I even came in 9 a.m. to 3 p.m. on Saturdays for open lab and supplemental instruction. At the end of the year, we had to complete part one of the national board exam that focuses on the basic sciences.

Diagram A shows a comparison of traditional medical school and chiropractic hours of study.

Chiropractic Student Hours	Class Description	Medical Student Hours
520	Anatomy	508
420	Physiology	326
271	Pathology	335
300	Chemistry	325
114	Bacteriology	130
370	Diagnosis	374
320	Neurology	112
217	X-ray	148
65	Psychiatry	144
65	Obstetrics and Gynecology	198
225	Orthopedics	156
2,887	Total Hours	2,756
1,598	Specialty Courses	1,492
4,485	Entire Total Hours	4,248

Diagram A

As you can see, there are slightly more classroom hours required by chiropractic education. Keep in mind, different schools have different curriculums and can vary slightly. However, overall, there's not a lot of difference in the total number of education and training hours between medical and chiropractic students, although the focus of those hours is different, which makes sense. I don't need much training in OB-GYN since I, hopefully, won't be delivering any babies.

In addition to going through extensive education, chiropractic students are also required to pass the National Board of Chiropractic Examiners (NBCE). These board exams are broken into four parts. Parts one through four are written, with part four and physiotherapy being more heavily weighted on diagnostic and practical skills. The more practical sections have several test stations complete with mock patients exhibiting certain signs and symptoms with positive clinical findings, their corresponding labs, x-rays, and history. There is then a panel of proctors asking questions with real-world applications about treatment, complications to treatment, and contraindications.

NBCE PART I BASIC SCIENCES:

General Anatomy

Spinal Anatomy

Physiology

Chemistry

Pathology

Microbiology

NBCE PART II CLINICAL SCIENCES:

General Diagnosis

Neuromusculoskeletal Diagnosis

Diagnostic Imaging

Principles Of Chiropractic

Chiropractic Practice

Associated Clinical Sciences

NBCE PART III CLINICAL AREAS:

Case History

Physical Examination

Neuromusculoskeletal Examination

Diagnostic Imaging

Clinical Laboratory and Special Studies

Diagnosis or Clinical Impression

Chiropractic Techniques

Supportive Interventions

Case Management

NBCE PHYSIOTHERAPY:

Thermotherapy

Ultrasound

Cryotherapy

Bracing/Orthotics

Taping

Cold Laser

Ultraviolet

Muscle Imbalances

Exercise Physiology

Muscle Rehabilitation

Neuromuscular Rehabilitation

Disorder-Specific Rehabilitation

NBCE PART IV PRACTICAL TESTING:

Diagnostic Imaging

Chiropractic Technique

Case Management

In the state of Illinois, if a chiropractor fails any part of the board a total of three times (for example, if they fail parts one and four and PT), they're done. They cannot practice in Illinois without further study.

That's a far more rigorous standard than what "real doctors" are held to—they don't have to be board certified to practice in Illinois. I have a good friend who is a practicing anesthesiologist at one of the best hospitals in Chicago, and he makes $450,000 a year. He is not board certified and cannot pass his boards—even though he's taken them several times.

How is it possible that chiropractic doctors have to be board certified but medical doctors don't? How is it possible that someone can perform surgery or anesthesiology or any other procedure that can result in death without being board certified? Of course, different states have different regulations and rules.

In Illinois, chiropractors are also required to complete 150 hours of continuing medical education every three years. A minimum of 60 hours of the required 150 hours needs to be in a formal category, which means classroom study conducted or endorsed by hospitals, specialty societies, facilities, or other organizations.

Given that, I'd argue that if anyone is a real doctor, chiropractors are certainly among them. There are several stereotypes about chiropractic that may prevent people from seeking treatment.

Perhaps the biggest differentiator between chiropractic doctors and medical doctors is their approach to treating patients. Biochemical problems such as hyperthyroidism and infections require a chemical solution, provided through medical doctors and prescription medications. Physical problems such as poor posture, back pain, neck pain, and headaches require a physical solution, provided by doctors of chiropractic. These chiropractors provide adjustments, corrective exercises, stretches, and other physical modalities to correct subluxation, or misalignment, of the spine. I understand that the goal of patients is most often to get out of pain, and that may be the extent of care they desire when they first present to my office.

As illustrated earlier, biochemical problems do often improve by correcting the subluxation, because that restores the master nervous system, allowing it to function correctly again.

Unfortunately, misinformation about what chiropractic is and what it does has led many people to avoid seeking preventative care, and that's too bad.

When I treat patients, my goal is to provide long-term relief. I want to make sure that five years from now, you're not back here with a bulging or herniated disc. I want to fight for you now, when a problem is an easy fix and won't require a lot of time and effort. I want to teach you things to do at home so that you can prevent the issue from becoming chronic and more serious.

COMMON MYTHS ABOUT CHIROPRACTIC

People have several stereotypes about chiropractic care that prevent them from seeking treatment, so I want to address those here. For example, a common myth I often hear is "If you go in once, you'll have to go in the rest of your life."

I understand that the goal of patients is most often to get out of pain, and that's the extent of care they desire when they come to my office.

Of course, if that's all they want, we can make it happen. We can rid the pain and part ways, but likely the patient will start experiencing similar pain again down the road. That's why I want people to think about chiropractic care similar to dental care—the prevention of decay.

Better health is a lifestyle, and chiropractic and alignment are pieces of that. If you put the best tires on a high-performance vehicle and they are not aligned properly, no matter how good the engine is, the car will not perform. Once you understand the value of regular chiropractic adjustments, you'll want to return regularly so that your spine doesn't degenerate, decay, or ache, and so your nerves don't become impinged. The subluxations (misalignment) will be detected and removed immediately before any permanent damage is done.

I'd like that to be something you choose to do—not something you're forced to do because your back requires the regular treatment.

Chiropractors do hope that once you come, you come forever. That way we're not perpetually chasing away pain; we're preventing it. We're changing your mindset so that you're focused away from being reactive to being more proactive when it comes to pain management, posture, and musculoskeletal health. That's not the same thing as hoping you come so that you have no choice but to come forever. Once you're there and understand how it works, you'll see that chiropractors come from an entirely different mindset than what's commonly perceived. Think dentistry.

I understand that once you're in pain, your priority is to make it stop, but the bigger picture goes beyond just eliminating your pain; it includes correcting the problem, teaching you how to stay out of pain, and changing the way you think about health, so that you're not popping high-cholesterol medication moments before pulling into the McDonald's drive-through. It's about helping you change your lifestyle so you don't have high cholesterol to begin with. (Do you think it's weird that a chiropractor would address your diet habits? That's another misconception. Read chapter 3 for more about that.)

It's our job as chiropractors to help you understand the value of coming to see us when you're not in pain, and educating you about the importance of preventative health care, dietary improvements, regular exercise, and spinal alignment to ensure your body functions optimally.

Another common myth I hear is that all we do is "crack backs." "Crack" implies breakage. We're not cracking anything. We're adjusting, we're aligning, we're manipulating, and about 60 percent of the time during that process you will hear a cavitation, or a pop or click, similar to the sound you hear when you crack your knuckles. The pop or click is the release of gas from the joint spaces. It is not in any way, shape, or form "cracking" anything. The pop, or cavitation, or click is not the adjustment itself; it's a by-product of alignment.

Adjustments can be done in many ways and are outlined in great detail in chapter 3. The adjustment can be as gentle as pressure or can require a more aggressive approach. These movements are designed to put a specific force in a specific direction to align the spine so your brain can communicate properly with your body. When we take the pressure off the nerve, the impulses flow freely and the body functions at a high level. Whichever procedure that is best for you should not be done haphazardly and should be explained in great detail before it is performed. As I explain each movement and what you can expect, most patients are pleasantly surprised and say, "That's it!" I am not really sure what people are expecting, but "yes, that's it."

Another common myth is this notion that chiropractors treat just back and neck pain. Sure, backs are a part—probably the most important part—of what we treat since your brain communicates with your body through the spine. However, chiropractors focus on much more than just your back. We are trained to align every joint in the body: ankles, shoulders, knees, and so on. As a certified chiropractic sports physician, I'd say a third of my practice centers around issues that aren't related to back pain—or at least the initial reason for seeking care is something other than back pain. Therefore, it's my job to educate patients on how various problems relate to proper spinal biomechanics.

There is also the misconception that chiropractic is expensive. Truthfully, it can be. Once you're already in pain and require a lot of treatments to get you out of that pain, the process can certainly be costly, as you'll often be required to come in multiple times a week to rectify a problem that's likely been ignored for years—just like if you were to put off filling a cavity. Root canals and advanced dental treatments that are a result of ignored cavities are often much more expensive than a simple filling.

Chiropractic care that is perceived to be expensive comes from the fact that it's typically not covered 100 percent by insurance companies. Nothing these days really is. At the dentist, getting a filling is expensive overall, but you pay only a small portion because insurance covers the majority of the cost. Even if you have to pay $50, you feel like you got a great deal because insurance covered the rest. There is no perceived value.

However, with chiropractic care, when you have to pay $60 because insurance doesn't cover anything, most people's eyes grow wide and they say, "I have to pay for the whole thing? That's ridiculous!" Even though it may be only $10 more, as in this example, it's still a big deal simply because insurance doesn't cover a penny.

The truth is, getting sick in the United States is expensive. Being treated for sickness is the number-one cause for bankruptcy and lost wages in this country. My advice to you is to invest in yourself with preventative care. You only get one body.

A patient's dad once told me, "It's really hard for me to pay for my son's care when I don't believe in chiropractic."

"You don't have to believe," I responded. "It's still going to work for him. Just give me thirty days. If after thirty days, you still don't think it's something you want to do, make that decision then."

Within two weeks, the young adult was a high scorer on his varsity basketball team for the first time in his life. He went from being benched with pain and weakness to being a top player in just two weeks!

"Since I've been under chiropractic care, I feel like I went from driving a bus to driving a Corvette," another patient stated.

Plenty of research supports that the benefits of chiropractic can be profound. For example, 90 percent of patients who see chiropractors have better pain outcomes than those who don't.[23] There are also noticeable benefits on blood pressure. Other research suggests that upper cervical vertebrae adjustments—which focus on the top two neck bones—are equal to taking two blood-pressure-lowering drugs simultaneously.[24]

Another incorrect perception is that chiropractic treatments can cause stroke. I find that this discussion becomes more political and emotional than it does scientific. The types of strokes referred to in these scare tactics are what we call *hemorrhagic strokes*. They're extremely rare and not to be confused with the much more common stroke called *ischemic strokes*. These types of strokes account for eight

23   C. M. Goertz et al., "Effects of usual medical care plus chiropractic care vs usual medical care alone on pain and disability among US service members with low back pain: a comparative effectiveness clinical trial," *Journal of the American Medical Association Network Open* 1, no. 1 (2018), https://doi.org/10.1001/jamanetworkopen.2018.0105.

24   University of Chicago Medical Center, "Special chiropractic adjustment lowers blood pressure," ScienceDaily, accessed September 1, 2018, www.sciencedaily.com/releases/2007/03/070315161129.htm.

out of ten strokes and are caused by blockages or clots. Neck adjustments cause no more stress to the arteries in the neck than any normal range of motion exercise. These hemorrhagic strokes can happen in the vertebrobasilar artery (VBA) and are so rare that they're difficult to even observe. According to one study, the odds of this type of stroke in the normal population, chiropractic patient or not, is 1 in 5.85 million people.[25] You have a better chance of being struck by lightning three times than having a VBA stroke. Because these types of strokes are so rare, they're challenging to research.

On the other hand, death rates from medications used to treat neck complaints (NSAIDs) are estimated to be around 16,500 per year.[26]

If I brush my teeth and then have a stroke, did the dental care cause the stroke? Of course not. Another study concludes you're just as likely to have a stroke after visiting a primary care physician as you are to have one after visiting a chiropractor.[27]

Healthier Illinois Natural First teamed up with the Illinois Chiropractic Society and ChiroUp to compile a patient information handout that summed it up best. From the studies mentioned they put into layman's terms as follows:

---

25   E. W. Church et al., "Systematic review and meta-analysis of chiro-practic care and cervical artery dissection: no evidence for causation," *Cureus* 8, no. 2 (February 16, 2016), https://doi.org/10.7759/cureus.498.

26   American Nutrition Association, "Deadly NSAIDS," *Nutrition Digest* 38, no. 2, http://americannutritionassociation.org/newsletter/deadly-nsaids.

27   J. D. Cassidy et al., "Risk of vertebrobasilar stroke and chiropractic care: results of a population-based case-control and case-crossover study," *Spine* 33, no. 4 (February 15, 2008), https://doi.org/10.1097/BRS.0b013e3181644600.

Study	Conclusion
J.D. Cassidy et al., "Risk of vertebrobasilar stroke and chiropractic care: results of a population-based case-control and case-crossover study," *Spine*	"No evidence of excess risk of stroke associated with chiropractic care to primary care."
Kosloff T.M. et al., "Chiropractic care and the risk of vertebrobasilar stroke," *Chiropractic & Manual Therapies*	"No significant association between stroke and chiropractic visits. Manipulation is an unlikely cause of stroke."
Church E.W. et al., "Systematic Review and Meta-analysis of Chiropractic Care and Cervical Artery Dissection," *Cureus*	"No causal link between chiropractic manipulation and Cervical Artery Dissection (stroke)."
Cassidy J.D. et al., "Risk of Carotid Stroke after Chiropractic Care: A Population-Based Case-Crossover Study," *Journal of Stroke and Cerebrovascular Diseases*	"No excess risk of stroke after chiropractic care."

Each study has concluded that chiropractic adjustments do not cause strokes. However, patients with symptoms such as neck pain and headaches are more likely to see a provider, such as a chiropractor. These symptoms could be from an impending stroke, but there is no causal relationship between the adjustment and the stroke.

Even though chiropractic neck adjustments are safe and effective, all necessary tests should be performed to ensure its effectiveness, as with any procedure. Your chances of dying from taking an Advil are significantly higher than dying from a visit to the chiropractor.

There's tangible proof that chiropractic care is safer than general medical treatments. And here it is: I've been in practice for nineteen years, and my malpractice insurance is less than $10,000 a year. This premium is after nineteen years of practice and tens of thousands of chiropractic adjustments. The average chiropractor has insurance rates that are far less than $10,000 a year. As mentioned in chapter 1, malpractice insurance for medical doctors is exorbitant because of the number of claims made. If chiropractors were causing strokes, our malpractice would be through the roof to settle those claims, and it's just not so.

The important thing to understand here is that the number of people who are happy and satisfied with complementary and alternative health care, including chiropractic, is much higher than those who are happy with their medical care. Statistics show, if you're using chiropractic care for worker's compensation recovery, your chances of going back to work are double compared to if you didn't use it.[28]

Let's go back to the myths—what feeds them? To be completely honest, I believe the American Medical Association (AMA) has had it out for chiropractors for a long time, and it's the body responsible for steering the conversation about chiropractic care. Chiropractors were put in jail in the 1950s and 1960s for practicing medicine without a license.

Things are changing between the AMA and the chiropractor community. No chiropractor is practicing medicine, and none of us want to. In turn, the AMA is beginning to realize that chiropractic care isn't going away—in fact it's the largest growing complementary and alternative health care in the country—so while they acknowledge it, they still compartmentalize it.

In addition to the AMA being partly responsible, there's also the pharmaceutical industry to consider, which has powerful lobbyists who disseminate information with any negative connotation they can muster.

To their luck, there's not much out there to refute that misinformation, as I mentioned in the previous chapter. My thirst for

---

28 S. P. Phelan et al., "An evaluation of medical and chiropractic provider utilization and costs: treating injured workers in North Carolina," *Journal of Manipulative and Physiological Therapeutics* 27 (September 2004): 442–8.

knowledge about chiropractic and natural health care, and any type of complementary and alternative medical treatment, was really stunted. The only way I could get any information was by taking chiropractors out to lunch so I could pick their brains.

To this day, even with the internet, there's little information and text about chiropractic from credible sources. Once you take a step back and look closely at what chiropractic really is, it makes logical sense. Why wouldn't you see a specialist for musculoskeletal problems?

Of course, who you go to matters. For instance, you wouldn't want a physician who is specialized in heart surgery to operate on the arteries or veins in your legs. There are other physicians, like a vascular surgeon in this case, who are more experienced and specialized in this area. Sometimes you encounter practitioners who want to be a jack-of-all-trades and master of none, which confuses patients.

The key thing to remember is that every discipline has its fair share of bad practitioners. The problem with chiropractors is that, for whatever reason, if you have a bad office experience, you'll discredit the entire profession. However, if you go to a primary care doctor and have a bad experience, you'll simply find a better one, right?

The same should apply to chiropractic. Find a chiropractor who listens to your concerns, who explains every procedure before it's done, and who cares for your health the way you do.

CHAPTER TAKEAWAYS:

- Gather information about what chiropractic really is. Do your homework—don't fall prey to rumors and misconceptions. It's your health. Educate yourself and ask questions.

- Chiropractors have a deeper medical education than most people realize. Their schooling is similar and comparable to traditional medical school—and exceeds it in areas where chiropractors specialize.

- Chiropractors don't treat cancer. They don't treat pneumonia. They study one major subject, so they're experts at what they do, because they do it every single day.

Chapter 3

WHAT CHIROPRACTIC REALLY IS

Chiro from *chiropractic* is Greek for *the hand,* which makes sense considering that chiropractic means to manipulate, typically by hand, any joint in the body to improve alignment and function.

In short, chiropractic is one thing and one thing only: the notion that misalignment or lack of movement in the spine can put pressure on nerves and cause dysfunction. The job of chiropractors is to relieve that spinal pressure and help your body perform optimally.

The practice of chiropractic is built on the premise that movement prevents degeneration. We know this is true of large joints in the body, which is why prolonged bed rest is

Varying degrees of luxation, or dislocation, can occur. It is widely accepted in the chiropractic community that *sub,* meaning partial, and *luxation,* meaning dislocation, are used to describe these rotations or impingements. For consistency in my practice and this book, subluxation is used to describe any partial dislocation. A full dislocation beyond normal range of motion (limit of anatomical integrity) would be termed a *dislocation.*

rarely used postsurgery; the quicker we get you moving, the better your results will be.

There are many ways chiropractic adjustments can occur, and many different techniques are used to achieve this goal. Not all techniques work best for all patients and all conditions, so it's important to find the one that works best for you.

Here is a list and brief descriptions of some of the techniques used:

- *Diversified Technique:* Probably the most widely used types of manipulation, and the most familiar to patients, this method entails a high-velocity, low-amplitude thrust that often results in a cavitation—the popping or clicking often associated with adjustments.

- *Extremity Manipulation/Adjusting:* This is the application of chiropractic manipulative therapy to joints other than the spine. The doctor may employ a variety of specific techniques to the shoulder, elbow, wrist, hip, knee, and other areas. Examples of conditions treated by extremity adjustments are plantar fasciitis, tennis elbow, impingement syndromes, and TMJ.

- *Activator Method:* This technique involves a spring-loaded handheld instrument that delivers the thrust, instead of the hands. This method is a great choice for patients who don't want manual manipulation or situations where manual manipulation would be inappropriate.

- *Thompson Technique:* This method uses a specialized table with moveable pieces that move in a specific direction to "distract" the joint and allow the adjustment to occur with less force. Cavitation may or may not be felt/heard.

- *Cox Flexion/Distraction:* This method also uses a table, in this case to pull the spine apart a bit to relieve pressure, and to flex the spine forward or side to side. This hands-on approach is often used with disc-related problems to increase the mobility of joints.

- *Gonstead Technique:* Another manual adjustment technique that focuses on the posterior to anterior thrust. Rotational adjustments are not utilized with this technique, and cavitation can be felt and heard.

- *NUCCA:* This method focuses on the vertebrae in the neck with a gentle touch on the first cervical vertebra.

- *Sacro Occipital Technique:* A low-force, slow-pressure technique usually leveraging gravity and the patient's body weight to correct misalignments. Triangular-shaped blocks are typically placed under the pelvis.

- *Webster Technique:* A specific chiropractic sacral analysis and diversified adjustment, with the goal of reducing the effects of sacral subluxation/sacroiliac (SI) joint dysfunction. In doing so, neuro-biomechanical function in the pelvis is facilitated. Sacral subluxation may contribute to difficult labor for the mother caused by inadequate uterine function, pelvic contraction, and baby malpresentation. Correction of sacral subluxation may have a positive effect on all of these causes of dystocia, or difficult births.

Although this isn't a comprehensive list of the many techniques chiropractors use, I've personally employed several of these to identify the best solution for each patient. Regardless of the technique used, the manipulation of a joint is termed an *adjustment*. A chiropractic adjustment is a common method for chiropractors to treat abnormally functioning joints. Adjustments involve the doctor applying very safe, specific, and controlled thrusts of varying speed and forces to the joints that are causing dysfunction and related pain. Adjustments push the involved joint beyond its normal range of motion into the paraphysiological space. This not only improves joint function but increases range of motion, making the likelihood of injury less.

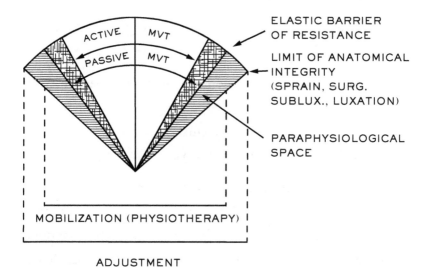

Physicians have mapped out that all the spinal nerves come from the brain and connect to all the organ systems, or tissues in your body, forming the information superhighway. The map showing where each spinal nerve connects to specific areas of your body is called the Meric System.

If the spinal column is not aligned properly, you'll experience dysfunction from the brain to that area of the body.

Another way to think of it is this: if you kink a hose, the water won't get to the nozzle. It's the same with your nerves. If a nerve is

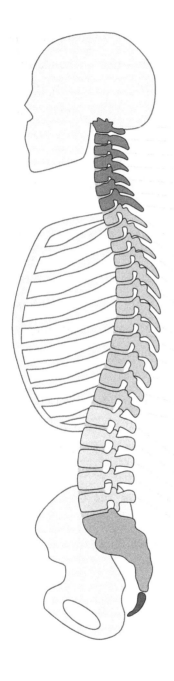

Cervical spine

C 1	Head - Brain - Inner and Middle Ears
C 2	Auditory Nerves - Sinuses - Eyes - Tongue
C 3	Teeth - Cheeks - Outer Ears
C 4	Nose - Mouth - Lips - Eustachian Tubes
C 5	Pharynx - Vocal Cords
C 6	Shoulders - Neck - Tonsils
C 7	Thyroids - Elbows

Thoracic spine

T 1	Trachea - Esophagus - Lower Arms - Fingers
T 2	Heart
T 3	Lungs - Chest - Breast
T 4	Gall Bladders
T 5	Liver - Blood Circulation - Solar Plexus
T 6	Stomach
T 7	Pancreas - Duodenum
T 8	Spleen
T 9	Adrenal Glands
T 10	Kidneys
T 11	Ureters
T 12	Small Intestines - Lymph Circulation

Lumbar spine

L 1	Large Intestines - Inguinal Region
L 2	Abdomen - Appendix - Upper Legs
L 3	Bladder - Sex Organs - Knees
L 4	Sciatic Nerves - Prostate Gland
L 5	Lower Legs - Feet

pinched or isn't working properly, something will be affected. Most of the time—but not always—the result is pain. Sometimes there are other symptoms. For example, if the information from your brain to your lungs isn't getting through correctly, there's a good chance your lungs won't function properly, and you'll suffer from a symptom, like asthma. If we can take the pressure off that nerve, it's possible your asthma symptoms will improve.

If there is pressure on a nerve that's affecting an organ system or tissue, the chance of it functioning at 100 percent is zero. It's impossible.

The problem becomes this: How do we trace exactly which vertebral segment is responsible for the symptom, whether it's back pain, asthma, allergies, reflux, or something else? That's a difficult task, which is why chiropractic is as much an art as it is a technique. Good chiropractors do all the necessary tests, exams, and imaging to determine what is causing your symptoms and then create a treatment plan to address those issues first.

For example, if you get headaches, we know based on clinical experience to look at the top cervical vertebra (called the *atlas*) and make sure it's positioned properly. In my experience, nine out of ten people who have headaches do not have the C1 vertebra in the proper position, which could create or increase the likelihood of these throbbing pains.

The art of chiropractic is knowing this information and, more importantly, educating people about it.

THE WORK OF A CHIROPRACTOR NEVER ENDS

The goal of the chiropractor—or what should be the goal of every chiropractor—is to correct the problem (subluxations), strengthen and stabilize the area, and teach patients ways to maintain that stability so they don't suffer again. Subsequently, as a result of the system being aligned and the spine not degenerating, patients will see an improvement in overall health and performance.

I've heard people say, "Well, my doctor says that degeneration is normal." Sure it is—only because people don't take care of themselves. They wait until they're in pain before they decide to have their spines fixed, and they only visit the chiropractor until the pain vanishes. Once it does, so does the patient.

However, that's not how chiropractic is meant to work. To be truly effective, it must be an ongoing process to help the patient maintain the health of their spine.

Think of your organs, bones, discs, etc., like you would the parts of a car. Once they experience significant wear and tear, they're less effective.

Similarly, once the discs in your spine are gone, they're gone forever. We can't rehydrate a disc that's degenerated. That's why your best—and really only—option is to avoid having the discs degenerate in the first place by keeping the spine aligned and maintained correctly so that when you bend, lift, or twist, your spine moves appropriately. Reduce the subluxations, increase range of motion, and improve imbibitions of blood and fluid to the disc spaces naturally.

That's what chiropractic is all about.

THE THREE COMPONENTS OF ILL HEALTH

Recovery from pain and dysfunction has three components: the physical, emotional, and chemical. I help patients align not just their spines but also their lifestyles in those three areas.

When patients come to me, typically they're most concerned about the physical component—their pain. That's what I focus on first. A physical problem requires a physical solution.

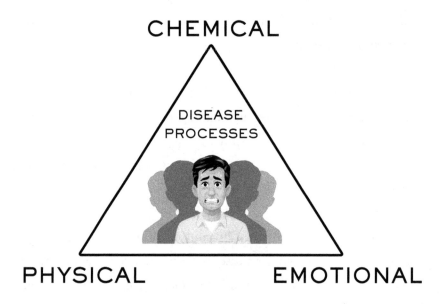

However, treatment during the physical component is more than just "cracking" someone's back—which we don't do at all, as explained in the earlier chapter and further in chapter 4. It involves studying exam results and x-rays and building a specific plan for each patient.

The chemical component includes everything you're putting into or on your body—food, drugs, alcohol, nicotine, etc.—that creates chemical reactions and affects the disease process you're experiencing. Obviously, if you're overweight, you're putting more pressure on your spine, which then promotes faster degeneration or misalignment. Also, if you're overweight, you're probably not exercising the way you should be because of the pain, which creates a vicious cycle.

This is why we address nutrition and food choices. Changing just a few habits can make a significant difference in someone's chemical health, and armed with the right information, it's easy to do. It is important we teach the patient to navigate all the misinformation and confusion in regard to the marketing of food.

Remember, those discs in your spine are fed by the things you put into your body. If you're smoking, your discs will degenerate faster. If you're not eating well, that will affect your spine. Even if you think you are eating healthy, today's fruits and vegetables aren't packed with nearly as many nutrients as they used to be, partly because we're overcultivating and using chemicals to grow a large portion of our crops. We are not only taking from the soil, but we're shipping more produce from other countries. This is why locally grown produce is more nutrient rich than those treated with chemicals or shipped from other countries. If your produce isn't nutrient rich, adding supplements to your diet is essential to ensure you're getting the vitamins and minerals you need.

In the average American diet, a few simple and healthful changes can make a huge difference in reducing the chemical component of the disease process. However, marketing for "healthy" foods and diets is extremely misleading to consumers.

During a recent talk on nutrition, I asked the crowd, "How many of you look at food labels?" I saw a lot more hands go up than I would have twenty years ago.

Then I asked, "What's the first thing you look at?" The majority of the people, of course, responded with *calories*, which isn't a bad thing.

The problem is, marketers know that's the first thing you look at, so they cut the serving sizes on their packaging. For instance, food manufacturers come up with hundred-calorie snack bags, misleading people to believe that because they're only a hundred calories, their snacks are healthy.

Of course, that's not true.

If you look at the food label on many popular snack bars, you'll notice a new trick that manufacturers are using. They are now changing one bar to two servings, which means the information you see is for only half the bar. However, rarely does someone eat half. Instead, they glance at the food label, feel happy about the calorie count, and devour the whole thing; what they miss is that they should multiply the nutrition information by two. This is just one example of how marketing and food labels fool us into becoming unhealthier every day.

Years ago, I became so frustrated with public nutrition misinformation, I had patients start keeping a food log, writing down everything they ate or drank for seven days. Then I had them highlight everything that's good for them. I am not exaggerating when I say, people were highlighting Diet Cokes, hundred-calorie processed snacks, and many other less-than-healthy items.

I'm not here to take away all the foods and treats you love. I live by the 80/20 rule. I want you doing things correctly *most* of the time. The times you want to indulge, you should. However, you have to know the difference between healthy and unhealthy eating. People get into trouble when they don't know the difference, or more importantly think they are eating well and, in actuality, they have a lot of room for improvement. (More on that in chapter 5.) Is this not what you imagined you'd be discussing with a chiropractor, or better yet, a real doctor?

Moving on to the emotional component of disease, let's think about an elderly couple who has been together a long time. Say one of them dies. Soon after, the other passes away without any known ailment. In those scenarios, the emotional component is a huge factor, because the surviving spouse was feeling depressed, frail, and vulnerable without the person they'd spent most of their life alongside.

Many books suggest that the mind is a very powerful thing. René Descartes is famously known for his saying, "I think, therefore I am."

I've read studies of people with terminal illnesses who fared much better once they started thinking positive thoughts or writing positive life experiences.

To be clear, I'm no expert in the emotional component, but I work closely with many types of clinical psychology professionals. The benefits of emotional support can have a profound impact on pain management and overall health. Most experts agree, medication is not step number one nor is dismissing the patient, indicating "it's all in your head."

A PRACTICAL SOLUTION FOR A RANGE OF ISSUES

Chiropractic care goes well beyond helping with back, neck, and hip pain. It's a solution for dealing with a lot of problems, all directly related to how well your spine is functioning or how well your pelvis and spine are functioning jointly, including the following:

- Ankle pain

- Arm pain, arm tingling, or arm numbness

- Carpal tunnel symptoms

- Chronic headaches

- Difficulty bending

- Difficulty sitting

- Fibromyalgia

- Hip pain, leg pain, leg numbness, or leg tingling

- Knee pain

- Lifting difficulties

- Neck injuries like whiplash

- Progressive weakness in one area

- Recurring joint pain, joint stiffness, or joint swelling

- Sciatica pain

- Scoliosis

- Shin splints

- Sleep problems due to neck or back pain

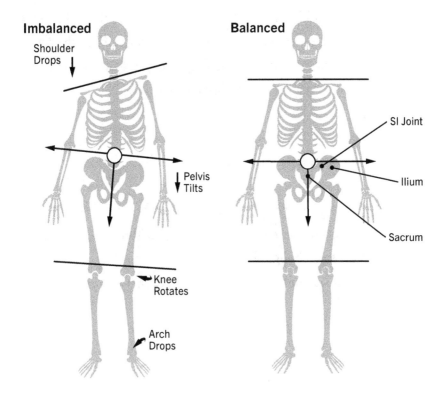

How can simple chiropractic solve all these problems? A lot of people have a hard time connecting how knee pain can diminish if you position the pelvis properly.

Think about the way your body is designed. Everything in your body is built off the spinal skeleton. The foundation of that spinal skeleton is what we call the *SI joint*. It's where the sacrum and the ilium—the uppermost and largest part of the hip bone—come together, creating your pelvis.

If the pelvis is not functioning properly, if it's out of position, the other side of the pelvis will compensate, with the result that one leg will be longer than the other. Therefore, every time someone with an out-of-alignment pelvis strikes the respective heel to the ground, it puts more pressure on that leg, causing knee pain, plantar fasciitis, not to mention ankle instability. Often when I explain that to a patient, they'll tell me one leg has always been longer than the other, so we'll take an x-ray of the pelvis and discover that it's the pelvis alignment causing the leg length discrepancy.

Putting the pelvis back in the proper position is the foundation for everything. Much like the foundation of a house. If the foundation is crooked, everything will compensate. I can't tell you how many times a patient with knee pain visited a medical doctor who wasn't able to diagnose the problem. In turn, the patient was simply instructed to stop running or stop playing golf. To me, that's as good as saying, "Just stop living life."

The better treatment is to examine the pelvis and tackle the problem.

In another case, a pregnant woman came to my office for counseling because her baby was breech. We did the Webster Technique, which is designed to loosen the pelvis to allow the baby to rotate so that it's sitting head first.

After four visits, the baby was in the proper position for a safe delivery. Not something you'd think about chiropractic for, huh?

Another example relates to the professional ballet dancer discussed in chapter 1. Her daughter had severe cerebral palsy and could not communicate. Although she was sixteen years old, she had the cognitive function of a six-year-old. The poor girl would sit in my waiting room and seize three or four times in the hour her mom was in my office. One day, her mom asked me, "Do you ever adjust children with cerebral palsy?"

I never had, but I would, I told her. I did my analysis, just like I would with any other patient. The girl had severe spinal misalignment, so I worked on adjusting her. After several treatments, she went from having dozens of seizures a day to one or two.

So that means I can cure seizures, right? No. No way. What I can do is take the pressure off a nerve, allowing the spine to function properly. And if that spine is contributing to whatever is affecting the patient, the symptoms will improve—the symptoms related to that nerve, anyway.

Chiropractic also helps improve posture, which is increasingly important in this age of mobile devices. Looking down while texting or slouching for hours on end is killing us. It's the new form of smoking.

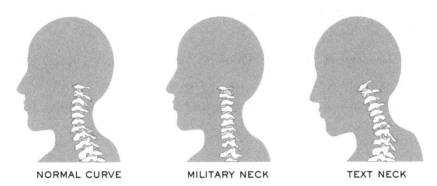

NORMAL CURVE   MILITARY NECK   TEXT NECK

Look around on a train or a bus, and you'll notice nearly every single person looking down at their phone for hours at a time. Heck, it's not uncommon to find two people sitting together in a restaurant, their heads bent toward their phones. That kind of posture leads to loss of your normal neck curve. We used to call it *military spine*, because it was thought to resemble people standing to attention; now we call it *text neck*. Text neck is known to be even worse because not only is it the loss of the normal cervical curve but the actual reversal in the opposite direction.

In the first five months of 2018, for example, I saw hundreds of patients with text neck—and only two or three with a normal curvature. That's a significant increase in the volume of patients who typically have a loss of curvature—particularly at a young age—perhaps because these patients never knew life without computers or cell phones.

Sleep posture is critical, as well. When you're lying on your back with your neck on a pillow, you are essentially putting your head in the same position as it is in when you're texting.

Sleeping on your side is even more damaging because it can cause sideways bending against the pillow.

Pillows exist for a reason: to make your bed look pretty. That's all.

To support normal curvature in your sleep, your chin should inch upward toward the ceiling, not downward toward your chest. I used to instruct patients to sleep on their backs to maintain this curvature. "Yeah, sure, doc," they'd say.

So now I've changed my approach. I tell them to do this simple exercise every night: Roll up two towels like a log and place one under the neck and the other under the lower back, lying face up for twenty minutes. Often, my patients tell me they fall asleep this way. Little do they know I'm training them to sleep on their backs. I have

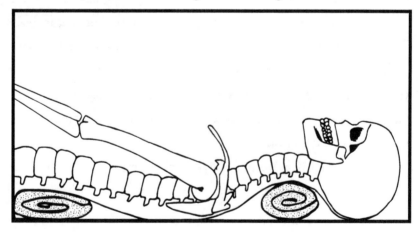

a video demonstration of this on my YouTube channel, DrIng-hamDC, under "Rolling and Using Towels.

And, yes, for those wondering, they have cervical pillows that can work equally as well—for $100 a pillow. Or you can do this free exercise. Not to mention, towels are found in every hotel room, so you don't have to travel with your special pillow.

A COURSE OF TREATMENT AT ADVANCED SPINE & SPORTS CARE

To help you understand how chiropractic works, we'll walk through a typical series of treatments I use in my clinic, Advanced Spine & Sports Care, a 3,700-square-foot multidisciplinary clinic located in Chicago, Illinois.

Generally, I don't begin adjustments on a first visit, because I want to study the patient's exam findings and x-rays in detail first. Adjustments start only after the study of the findings is complete, and I determine the adjustments are safe and will be effective. We do, however, have a consultation with the patient about why they're there, and I collect pertinent x-rays, MRIs, blood work, and other medical information that allows me to formulate a logical treatment plan. Also, we'll often do some passive physical therapy for pain control, such as interferential current or intersegmental traction. Interferential current, or some form of muscle stimulation, is utilized to penetrate the muscle and drive inflammation from the area. Intersegmental traction is a type of traction the patients love. It feels great, but more importantly it opens up the disc spaces and helps nourish the disc.

"Why do you want the lab results from my blood work?" patients often wonder. For two reasons: One, I want the patient's complete medical file so that it is comprehensive and so that I can be an advocate for them. Two, most lab work is interpreted by computers nowadays and is measured against a generalized set of standards. I want to apply the patient's results against their unique physiology.

Hundreds of patients come in every year and report that they've already had x-rays taken, and the results were normal. However, when I do a basic measurement of their spine and curvature, I find that it's not normal. Or the x-rays taken in the conventional medical office were done with the patient lying down, which doesn't provide an accurate depiction of what is going on when gravity is applied to the spinal posture while standing.

On the second visit, a report of findings is completed. I personally go through each x-ray with them. We talk about what's wrong, the anticipated adjustment process, and more importantly, whether I can help with the problem. If I can't, I'll try to find someone who can. If I've determined that I can help, I schedule three consecutive visits. These visits allow me to monitor the patient closely and formulate the best course of treatment. This is an important point. Sometimes a patient comes in and tells me, "I tried chiropractic and it didn't help!" Well, "trying chiropractic" does not mean going for two or three visits in the span of a month and then stopping when nothing's changed. Most often, problems take several years to develop, so it can take time for the body to respond to care.

Most new patients are curious about how long treatment will take and how much it will cost. That's why another thing we have mastered is a mini-financial consultation, which includes verifying their insurance coverage and how much they'll have to pay out of pocket each session.

That second visit is also when the patient's first adjustment takes place. Patients can't really see what I'm doing when I'm aligning them, so naturally, they're a little apprehensive. I try to eliminate that fear by explaining exactly what I'll do before I do it, so the patient knows exactly what to expect, from my hand placement to breathing instructions.

The first three adjustments are probably the most important because they help me determine the best course of treatment. I like to keep those first three adjustments close together and variables as constant as possible throughout these visits. For instance, if you work out, I want you to keep working out. If you don't, I don't want you to start. I want to see how your body responds to care when you are doing what's normal for you.

On the third adjustment, or fourth visit, I go over the four-phase approach to functional health recovery and how long I expect each phase to last, and then bring in my financial coordinator, who goes over the cost in its entirety. This visit's financial consultation is different from the miniconsult done on day two because it lays out the four-phase approach and the cost for each phase in one large transparent presentation. Advanced Spine & Sports Care's financial coordinator's sole responsibility is walking patients through the pitfalls of insurance coverage.

From there on, patients come in as often as necessary for their treatment plan to be effective. Along the way, we track progress to ensure we're getting the results desired. My office does some combination of passive physical therapy—ultrasound, some form of electrical stimulation, heat, or ice—and then the actual chiropractic manipulation.

Depending on how much pain the patient is in, we start neuromuscular reeducation as soon as practically possible. This reeducation helps retrain the brain and the muscles to work together. Postural muscles may have never had good pathways to begin with if poor posture began at an early age. This lack of neuromuscular function is illustrated when patients admit, "It hurts to sit up straight" or "My back and neck get too tired with proper posture."

This reeducation process starts simply. We'll have the patient sit on a wobble board so their pelvis is unstable and they're forced to continuously correct their posture by exercising their muscles. This reeducation of muscle and nervous system function is critical for complete and maximized recovery.

When they reach the point where the pain is gone or much improved, we look into the next phase of care, tracking the progress and the expectations through that phase (again, more on that in chapter 5). At that point, correction in the spine begins. The focus of care becomes on health and wellness and less on pain.

During the strengthening phase of care, passive physical therapy is discontinued, and we start primarily focusing on active therapy. By this point, my hope is that patients are doing the sleep exercise and maybe falling asleep on their backs occasionally.

If there's one thing you should know, it's this: chiropractic is not a thirty-second fix. It's a lifestyle, an alternative way of thinking. That's too much to process for some people, so I start by focusing on alleviating the back pain, neck pain, headaches— or whatever else they come in for. Then, gradually, I lead them down the path to better health and an improved lifestyle through chiropractic. Treat symptoms locally, but rehabilitate globally.

UNDERSTANDING THE POWER OF CHIROPRACTIC

One day, a thirty-six-year-old man, Ray, came into my office with serious back pain. He'd been injured at work, and his place of employment sent him to a workers' compensation doctor. That doctor put him on medication, then stronger medication, and then six weeks of physical therapy.

All of that was of no help.

As a result, the doctor gave him three steroid injections. The first was slightly helpful, the second was less helpful, and the third was not helpful at all.

In fact, Ray was slightly worse at the end of that round of treatment than when he'd first started.

The workers' comp doctor sent him to an orthopedist, who recommended an MRI. From the MRI, the doctors determined that Ray had a series of bulging discs—L4, L5, and S1—and they recommended a lumbar fusion surgery.

Before the surgery, Ray came to me for a consultation. "Give me thirty days," I told him.

Because workers' compensation would not pay for my services, coming to me was a tough decision for him. He had the option of getting cut open for free or paying out of pocket to try something less invasive. If my treatment didn't work, he could always get the surgery later, I reminded him.

Initially, anyone in that situation would think that if the treatment were successful, workers' compensation would cover it, right?

Unfortunately, that's not the way it works. The unwillingness of workers' compensation to cover chiropractic services isn't a reflection of our effectiveness; rather, it's a testament to their desire to seek more traditional—and more profitable—courses.

Ray agreed to try chiropractic treatments for a month, during which time he came in for twelve adjustments.

At the end of the month, he was back at work—with no symptoms whatsoever.

Ray's situation is not an unusual one. Yes, there are times when surgery is necessary—such as when bowel and bladder function is affected, or when nerves are impinged and cause muscle atrophy. However, if you go in and surgically fuse those levels together and the surgery doesn't help, your options for any future treatments would be extremely limited. And often it doesn't work; they call it *failed back surgery syndrome*. Understand that this is an actual diagnosis, and it's happening way more frequently than you may realize.

When we're in the phase of examining x-rays, we look for mis-alignment, both of the pelvis and of the spine. If there is a problem with general alignment, I can help you. If there isn't, surgery may be the answer.

One of the issues chiropractors can undoubtedly help with is a bulging disc. However, most people don't know what those are and end up misusing the term.

The inside of the disc is called the *nucleus pulposus*. This portion takes a majority of the downward compression when you walk, run, or jump. The outer circle of the disc is less elastic, less pliable. It takes less of the downward compression of your spine when you're walking or sitting.

A bulging disc occurs when the nucleus pulposus bulges outside of its normal confines. It doesn't necessarily mean that there's nerve impingement. A herniation means that the outer ring of the disc space has now extruded so that the inside of the disc is outside the

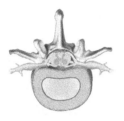

NORMAL DISC

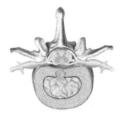

BULGING DISC

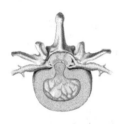

CENTRAL HERNIATED DISC

normal confines of the disc space (prolapsed), sometimes putting pressure on a nerve, other times narrowing, or stenosing, the spinal canal.

People often hear that they have spinal stenosis, but that doesn't necessarily mean that the disc is the problem. Inflammation as a result of an injury can stenose the spinal cord. Inflamed muscle can stenose the spinal cord. Even movement of spinal bone can stenose the spinal cord.

If we can train the body not to create that inflammation in the first place by retraining muscles and applying proper spinal alignment, we can relieve the pressure on the nerve and the pain that pressure creates.

Think of it this way: if someone has a sprained ankle and doesn't do anything about it, letting it heal on its own, the chances of that ankle spraining again approaches 100 percent. If you sprain it once, the chances you'll do it again are near guaranteed—especially for athletes.

The same goes for just about any joint in your body. The idea that the pain will go away or that because the joint stopped hurting it's healed is a faulty thought process. It's just a matter of time before the inflammation, or the bone, or the disc, or whatever it is, finds the nerve again, and then you're right back to where you started, and often the symptoms are more severe. For every day that pain is present, it is one step closer to becoming permanent.

On the other hand, if the bulging disc is treated properly and if it's rehabbed correctly, we can teach your body that it's not an injury and that the body does not need to respond with inflammation. Because the problem may have been present for a long time and the body is used to responding with inflammation, convincing it that this isn't somewhere it needs to induce inflammation can be challenging and may take several months.

I've seen patients with sixteen-millimeter (roughly half an inch) herniations who are pain free. Then I've seen people with two-millimeter herniations who can't get out of bed. That's why, in my opinion, it really is back to the basics. It's looking at how your body performs. It's looking at the joint function of the spine, and more importantly, it's about making sure it's working properly—because frequently there's some problem with general alignment. Is that always the cause of the pain? No. But a very high percentage of the time, it is. From my twenty years of clinical experience, it seems that half of the people with herniations don't even know they have them.

My position is: let's look at the easiest thing to fix, which is the inflammation caused by the herniation or injury, and the fact that the bone could be putting pressure on the nerve (reduce the subluxations). Those are easy fixes. We don't have to cut you open. There are no drugs. There is no surgery. We use our hands and manipulate the spine. Adjust the diet as well, and these changes will improve the physical and chemical components of the patient's condition.

Let's make sure alignment isn't the problem before we start cutting things away or fusing discs and then discovering that those didn't help because we weren't tackling the right problem. You can't undo surgery, but you can explore alternative options before you decide to get surgery.

Lori, a fifty-two-year-old woman, came to my office four years ago for a consult because she had back pain. I discovered she had spinal alignment problems. Her insurance didn't cover my services, and she lived too far away, so she ended up going to a surgeon who fused three of her neck vertebrae together.

Recently she came to see me again, this time in tears. "I'm ready to listen to you now," she said.

"Okay," I said. "Tell me about your past medical history."

"I had fusion surgery two years ago, and I'm in worse shape than I was when I came to you."

I looked at her, shocked, and said, "Okay, let me request your surgical records, update your file, and see what I can do to help.

What I found was that she'd had three vertebrae fused—at that point, there was nothing I could do. I could take care of the ones below and above those, but I can't manipulate fused vertebrae, not to mention the numerous rods, screws, and hardware she now had in the spine.

We all have excuses, but stop making them. Get the problem taken care of, and for God's sake, get second, third, and fourth opinions if you have to before you let someone cut you open.

CHAPTER TAKEAWAYS:

- Chiropractic is a natural health care alternative that can manage common musculoskeletal complaints.

- Your chiropractor can be a portal-of-entry doctor who can make referrals when appropriate.

- Chiropractic does not cure anything; it allows your body to heal itself when the communication system between your brain and body is restored and working optimally.

Chapter 4

CHIROPRACTIC FIRST

That ballet dancer's death still haunts me. I know I should have done more, should have explained—insisted—to her the drawbacks and dangers of relying on opioids to numb her pain.

I'm not meek anymore. Now I'm borderline obnoxious about preaching the benefits of chiropractic over pain meds and surgery—and I've seen the proof of those benefits throughout my life, both professionally and personally.

I've been getting regular spinal adjustments since I was six years old. Today, I'm forty-six. I look at other people my age who have chronic back and neck problems. I've never had those problems. I've run marathons and suffered sports injuries, so I know from a physical injury perspective how much chiropractic care has helped me and kept me well. I've never needed to take pain meds or use other medical approaches to deal with musculoskeletal pain—not even after I was in a bad car accident. I had rolled my truck and was literally dangling from my seat belt. In the emergency room, I was diagnosed with a concussion, whiplash, and several abrasions from the shattered windows of the truck. The doctors prescribed me pain meds and sent me on my way. However, rather than take the pills, my chiropractor evaluated and treated me for the injuries I sustained. I can't imagine doing anything other than going to the chiropractor.

And there's plenty of statistical and anecdotal evidence that shows these effects aren't confined to me.

CHOOSING AN EFFECTIVE, MORE ECONOMICAL, LESS INVASIVE ALTERNATIVE

In my practice, I've seen—hundreds of times—just how powerful chiropractic has been in improving the quality of life for people who have certain ailments. It helps with neck and back pain, sure, but the benefits extend beyond just those.

For instance, take the impact that chiropractic care can have on children. Since infants can't talk, we don't get all the confusion with them saying one thing but meaning another. We go by how they physically react. They either have an ear infection, or they don't. They're either colicky, or they're not. They either have reflux, or they don't. They can't exaggerate or minimize problems.

Those babies have helped me learn just how impactful an adjustment can be to the body as a whole, affecting even seemingly unrelated problems within it.

My nephew, for example, had recurring ear infections. My sister had been taking him to the chiropractor just once a month, which really isn't enough to maintain optimal benefits, particularly for a toddler learning to walk. Imagine all the trauma to the developing body from the bumps and bruises of learning these new skills. I recommended that she talk to the chiropractor and take him more often. When she did, the earaches disappeared. (Remember the information highway we talked about?) I've seen the same phenomenon with other infants, and also with infants who have reflux.

When you're able to reduce a child's reflux or ear infections, you're changing the course of their lives—those kids are happier, and their parents are happier.

Asthma is another chronic issue I often see in my practice. To be clear, I don't cure asthma, reflux, or earaches, but I can tell you that numerous patients who were seeing me for headaches and back or neck pain would say to me, "Hey, doc, I know this sounds crazy, but I haven't had to use my inhaler since I started coming to you." Listen, if you can get your brain to communicate clearly, through releasing pressure on spinal nerves, with the organs and systems in your body, those tissues will function better.

A new report from the CDC shows by helping overweight and obese patients lose weight, chiropractors can contribute to the prevention of cancer. The study found that 50 percent of cancers in men and 24 percent of cancers in women in the United States were associated with overweight and obesity.[29] Because such a high percentage of young adults are overweight, doctors of chiropractic can play a key role in aiding patients with this problem by offering an alternative to fad diets and potentially harmful weight-loss drugs and surgeries. Chiropractic doctors study nutrition, fitness, and healthy eating at a level most medical doctors do not.

Beyond that, science- and evidence-based research supports the idea that chiropractic promotes an overall healthier life. A report in the journal *Spine* concluded that "SMT (spinal manipulation therapy) is effective for the treatment of chronic nonspecific LBP

---

29 "Cancers associated with overweight and obesity make up 40 percent of cancers diagnosed in the United States," Centers for Disease Control and Prevention (October 3, 2017).

(low back pain)."[30] The study suggests that regular maintenance spinal manipulation, even after initial treatment and symptoms have subsided, can provide long-term benefits.

Another study, published in the *Journal of Occupational and Environmental Medicine*, found that among 894 injured workers who were observed for a year, those who went through physical therapy treatment had the highest instance of reinjured workers. The second highest was among those who received standard medical treatment (or no treatment at all). "The lowest incidence of repeat injury was found among those workers who had received chiropractic maintenance care," the report states.[31]

Analysis of Medicare claims revealed a strong inverse relationship between the supply of chiropractors/chiropractic care and opioid prescriptions.[32]

In an excellent example of the kind of comparative effectiveness research needed to distinguish the competing treatment approaches, researchers in Alberta, Canada, studied the relative costs and benefits of lumbar (lower back) microdiscectomy—a minimally invasive surgical procedure for patients with a herniated lumbar disc—and chiropractic spinal manipulation for patients with low back pain and sciatica associated with lumbar disc herniation for whom usual medical care had failed. As stated earlier, a herniation occurs when

---

30 M. K. Senna and S. A. Machaly, "Does maintained spinal manipulation therapy for chronic nonspecific low back pain result in better long-term outcome?" *Spine* 36, no. 18 (August 15, 2011): 1427–37.

31 Manuel Cifuentes, Joanna Willetts, and Radoslaw Wasiak, "Health maintenance care in work-related low back pain and its association with disability recurrence," *Journal of Occupational and Environmental Medicine* 53, no. 4 (April 2011): 396–404.

32 William B. Weeks and Christine M. Goertz, "Cross-sectional analysis of per capita supply of doctors of chiropractic and opioid use in younger Medicare beneficiaries," *Journal of Manipulative and Physiological Therapeutics* 39, no. 4 (May 2016): 263–266.

a tear in the outer, fibrous ring of an intervertebral disc allows the soft, central portion of the disc to bulge out beyond the damaged outer rings, causing sensitivity and irritation. The results of this research were dramatic: 60 percent of patients with sciatica—pain that radiates along the path of the sciatic nerve, which branches from the lower back through the hips and buttocks and down each leg—benefited from spinal manipulation to the same degree as if they had undergone surgical intervention, and at a far lower cost.

The economic implications of these findings are far reaching. In the United States, at least two hundred thousand microdiscectomies are performed annually, at a direct cost of $5 billion, or $25,000 per procedure. Preventing 60 percent of these surgeries would mean a reduction of $3 billion annually. In the Canadian study, patients receiving chiropractic care averaged twenty-one visits during the course of their care. If a cost of $100 per patient visit is assumed for the care provided by the chiropractor, then the total cost per patient is $2,100, yielding per-patient savings of $22,900, or $2.75 billion annually.[33]

---

33 G. McMorland et al., "Manipulation or microdiscectomy for sciatica? A prospective randomized clinical study," *Journal of Manipulative Physiological Therapy* 33, no. 8 (October 2010): 576–584.

CHIROPRACTIC: A TREATMENT THAT MAKES NEUROLOGICAL SENSE

Why does chiropractic work? In simple terms, every system, tissue, and organ in your body is innervated by nerves. All the spinal nerves come from the brain to the organ, system, or tissue through the spine. That is the "information superhighway" mentioned previously.

There are twenty-four movable vertebrae in your spine. Between those bones are soft discs that allow you to bend, lift, or twist. Spinal nerves exit out of tiny holes between each of the vertebrae at the disc level. If the spine is stuck or not moving properly, it can put pressure on a nerve. The disc can start to die or degenerate due to the lack of movement. Left untreated, this can lead to bulging discs, herniated discs, or degenerative disc disease.

In the case of asthma, for example, if the information highway from your brain to your lungs isn't functioning correctly, how can your lungs function correctly? They can't.

If I can take the pressure off the nerve, the communication from the lungs to the brain can be reestablished. And if the communication between the brain and your lungs is improved, is there a chance that the symptom you're experiencing—in this example, asthma—will be improved? That certainly seems logical, right?

To illustrate this point, I use a diagram called the brain/body diagram:

BRAIN/BODY DIAGRAM

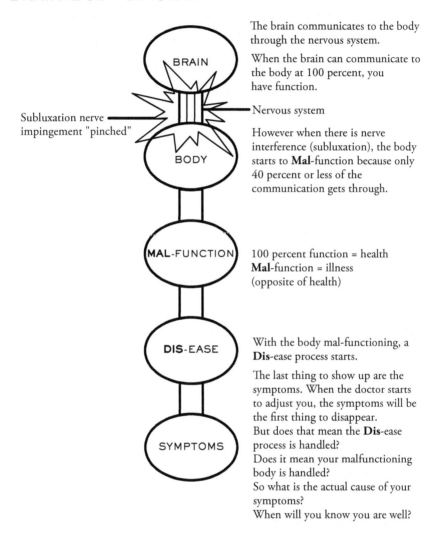

The brain communicates to the body through the nervous system.

When the brain can communicate to the body at 100 percent, you have function.

However when there is nerve interference (subluxation), the body starts to **Mal**-function because only 40 percent or less of the communication gets through.

100 percent function = health
Mal-function = illness
(opposite of health)

With the body mal-functioning, a **Dis**-ease process starts.

The last thing to show up are the symptoms. When the doctor starts to adjust you, the symptoms will be the first thing to disappear. But does that mean the **Dis**-ease process is handled? Does it mean your malfunctioning body is handled? So what is the actual cause of your symptoms? When will you know you are well?

It starts with the noodle-like, complex organ housed in your skull—your brain. The brain is connected to every organ, system, and tissue in your body by bundles of fibers called *nerves*. When this communication is functioning at 100 percent, your body is in a state of homeostasis or ease. If these nerves become impinged—

commonly called *pinched*—by too much pressure from surrounding bones, inflammation, discs, muscles, or tendons, there is pain, or there is lack of flow from the brain to the part of the body that the nerve supplies, and we say there's mal-function. This mal-function then leads to a state of dis-ease. Only after this mal-function and dis-ease are left untreated do you experience the symptom—but it's much like how the oil light in your car functions—once it turns on, you already have big problems to face.

Going back to the basic concepts of physiology and anatomy, I'll use a vehicle as an example. I could take the best high-performance vehicle, but if the wheels are misaligned, that car is not going to perform the way it's meant to—just as you are not going to perform your best if your spine is misaligned.

Chiropractic treatment for pain and biomechanical disorders is actually a widely accepted idea. However, poor education among doctors and consumers coupled with insurance companies writing chiropractic treatment off as an "elective modality" makes it seem less of a practical, affordable option.

Chiropractic, however, is not elective. It's essential to a healthy body and great quality of life.

TECHNOLOGY'S INFLUENCE

With computers, handheld devices, and texting now a daily part of life, the average young adult's posture is worsening, leading to more misalignment. It doesn't take a brain surgeon to notice that society is suddenly walking around more hunched over than before from texting on that cell phone all day. Couple that with sitting at a computer eight hours a day, and we are looking more and more like grandma at an earlier and earlier age. Next time you are at a restaurant, take a moment to look around. I've noticed as many as four people sitting less than three feet from each other at a table and all of them are engaged with their devices. I have a friend who even suggests that everyone put their cell phones in the middle of the table and the first one to touch their phone has to buy dinner. Our goal, from a chiropractic perspective, is to prevent those poor posture habits, as well as future problems, by aligning the spine properly and teaching you how to keep it that way.

If we don't prevent misalignments, you'll experience pain, which is the last thing to occur once malfunction and disease have already begun. Of course, people often ignore the pain until they have to crawl into the office, seeking chiropractic treatment as a last-ditch effort. That's the medical model our health care system is based on—"sick care," where you wait until you're sick before you take action. By that point, my job—or the job of any health care provider—is much more difficult than if you had come to me proactively.

We must view body and health care from a different perspective and change that paradigm. As stated previously, we should adopt a more dental-based model; I brush and floss and visit the dentist twice a year to prevent my teeth from decaying. If I wait until I'm in pain, it likely means I already have cavities and my tooth or teeth have died or degenerated. We need to apply that same model in health care, where we practice preventive measures rather than reactive tactics.

The benefits of a preventive approach extend beyond just personal health—they promote better community health. When we take advantage of all that chiropractic care can offer, we can change the paradigm and get out from underneath the health care crisis we discussed previously.

How? Let's take a look.

SAVING DOLLARS WITH THE RIGHT CARE

A 2018 review of Medicare data from New Hampshire showed that recipients of chiropractic services had a 55 percent lower likelihood of filling an opioid prescription.[34] Are there other variables in there? Sure. However, that decrease is significant and a strong indication that chiropractic treatments can help combat the opioid addiction issue.

Additionally, the research concluded that the average total charges for clinical services were significantly lower for recipients of chiropractic care compared to nonrecipients.

In a study from 2010, BlueCross BlueShield of Tennessee examined eighty-five thousand subscribers who had equal access to chiropractors and medical care—same copay and same cost per visit/treatment. Researchers found that the cost of care for low back pain with a chiropractic doctor was 40 percent lower than with a medical doctor.[35]

According to the analysis, if those subscribers had first visited a chiropractor, BlueCross BlueShield would have saved $2.3 million over the lifetime of the study.[25]

---

34   J. M. Whedon et al., "Association between utilization of chiropractic services for treatment of low-back pain and use of prescription opioids," *Journal of Alternative and Complementary Medicine* 24, no. 6 (June 2018): 552–556. https://doi.org/10.1089/acm.2017.0131.

35   R. L. Liliedahl et al., "Cost of care for common back pain conditions initiated with chiropractic doctor vs medical doctor/doctor of osteopathy as first physician: experience of one Tennessee-based general health insurer," *Journal of Manipulative and Physiological Therapeutics* 33, no. 9 (November–December 2010): 640–3. https://doi.org/10.1016/j.jmpt.2010.08.018.

If we can save money on insurance costs, we might be able to bring down overall health care costs, making medical care more affordable for everyone.

As copayments and coinsurance costs continue to rise, chiropractic treatments are becoming increasingly important for individuals—and more affordable. As mentioned in chapter 1, people are spending hundreds of thousands of dollars on surgeries they don't need or that have less than a 50 percent chance of being beneficial. For $100,000, you can get a lifetime of chiropractic care.

My initial consult, which includes x-rays, is often less than a patient's deductible, possibly less than what you're paying for your copayment—about the cost of a dinner for two or a monthly gym membership. And that's my entire cost. There are no surprises. No hospital fees. You're not going to get a bill for $3,000 later because your insurance didn't cover something it told you it would.

Then there's the issue of impersonal care most people receive through traditional health care physicians, leaving patients feeling like a number. People have often coached me to become less available to my patients. However, to this day, I give my personal email address to every patient and check it twice a day, every day, answering all correspondences I receive.

THE SIGNIFICANT AND DIVERSIFIED ROLE OF A CHIROPRACTOR

In today's health care landscape, chiropractors are more than just "back doctors." We are portal-of-entry providers for all your health care needs.

Think of it like finding a good OB-GYN, dentist, or primary care physician whom you visit regularly for preventative care. I'm a primary care physician for a lot of my patients, and I'm okay with that. I think that's the way it should be, because my primary care answers are going to be a heck of a lot more cost effective, as well as a heck of a lot less damning to your body than what traditional medicine offers—treatments that mask more and fix less.

I believe the future of chiropractic care will be just that—the chiropractor will be a member of the health care team who takes time to educate you on preventative measures.

However, until then, we need to educate our patients—and more importantly, educate our frontline physicians and medical specialists—on how chiropractic care can benefit both patients and the health care crisis. Thomas Edison said, "The doctor of the future will give no medicine." The doctor of the future is here.

NOT A ONE-SIZE-FITS-ALL SOLUTION

Not all back pain is musculoskeletal related, and I understand that; every chiropractor is trained to understand that. There are other issues that can cause low back pain: kidney stones and abdominal dysfunction are among the possible diagnoses. Chiropractic doctors, however, are trained to identify such situations and, when needed, refer patients for the care they need.

While I can't fix everyone, I'm able to help most people by examining their x-rays and lab work to diagnose the underlying issue. Luckily, most of the time, the problem is something that can be corrected pretty quickly, and I'm able to help educate people about ways to prevent a similar problem in the future.

Unfortunately, today, most of my treatments are centered around helping patients overcome pain and correcting the problem. Only after that happens am I able to actually stabilize and strengthen the area, and educate the patient about the root cause so they don't reinjure themselves.

My hope is to never let patients even get to the pain part or the crisis care. I want to teach you what to do so that you're seeing your chiropractor only for maintenance care—all for the investment of thirty minutes and about $60 per appointment.

That's the value chiropractic can bring to modern medicine and the way it can create a paradigm shift.

The current system isn't working. Changing mindsets is not easy, but it's the only way we can weaken, halt, and reverse the crisis we are currently in. With our generation, we might already be too late, but that doesn't mean we can't try for generations to come.

CHAPTER TAKEAWAYS

- Treatment for lower back pain initiated by a chiropractic doctor is 40 percent less expensive than when initiated by a medical doctor.

- Patients who visit a chiropractor have a 55 percent lower chance of filling a prescription for opioids.

- Patients who seek chiropractic care often experience relief of symptoms they did not associate with chiropractic care.

Chapter 5

THE REVOLUTIONARY FOUR-STAGE APPROACH TO FUNCTIONAL HEALTH RECOVERY

You've probably seen it happen in a movie or television show: a man or woman goes to a chiropractic clinic for an adjustment. Without warning, the chiropractor sneaks up on them and cracks their back, surprising the victim and usually leaving them sorer and stiffer than before.

In reality, some chiropractors do operate that way, but they're in the minority, and they're not the doctors I would recommend to my friends and family. A surprise approach is not the way to achieve the best patient outcome.

One patient told me that her last chiropractor snuck up behind her and adjusted her neck. "It scared me to death," she said.

To be fair, I'm not sure if that's what actually happened, but even if that's her perception of what occurred, it means the chiropractor did a poor job of communicating and setting expectations. Chiropractic isn't meant to be a party trick. It's not a "hey-look-over-there" moment followed by a swift manipulation while your guard is down.

A bad chiropractic procedure often means there was a lack of communication either from doctor to patient or patient to doctor. It's just as important that the chiropractor understand what's ailing you as it is for you to understand what they're going to do to correct your problem.

Before I adjust anyone, I do a series of necessary tests to ensure the patient is a good candidate for the treatment; that's a very important part of chiropractic care. If I'm at a barbecue and someone asks, "Hey, can I have an adjustment?" or "Hey, I've got this neck pain. Can you adjust it right here for me?" I'm going to educate on why this may not be the best course of action.

Chiropractic must be done correctly, or it can have adverse consequences.

However, people don't know much about chiropractic, and they don't know what to expect, so it's up to the chiropractor to fill in the blanks and educate them.

Your chiropractor should speak with you, teach you what's wrong, what's the problem, and how chiropractic can help. We want you to be relaxed, only because if you're stiff and trying to protect the area being aligned, you could create a negative response. However, there are techniques to help you relax, such as by having you wiggle your toes or think of a positive place like a warm, sunny beach.

Even then, your chiropractor should explain to you what they're going to do before they do it. For instance, I want my patients to know what to expect and what that would sound like because it's the sounds more than anything that people tend to be apprehensive about.

Lack of communication can lead to other problems too. For example, people frequently say, "After my adjustment, I hurt worse than when I went in." That's not uncommon; about 10 percent of the population experiences soreness after their first few adjustments. Generally, that's a result of trying to correct too much too soon. The doctor's heart might be in the right place because they may be trying to fix as much as possible during each visit, but on the other end, the patient leaves feeling miserable.

Chiropractors should talk to patients about the possibility of being sore. They should explain that, much like when an orthodontist tightens braces, there can be soreness for a day or two, so the patient shouldn't be alarmed. They should instruct them to place ice on the soreness and inform the chiropractor of it during the next visit.

I've adjusted people who felt like the human equivalent of trying to adjust a brick wall. I knew they would be sore that night, so I made sure to tell them to expect that soreness. If I didn't, they'd think I made them worse or, worse yet, that chiropractic didn't work.

It's important to educate and teach people what to expect, whether it be positive or negative. That's why the consultation is the most important part of the exam. People usually hesitate to speak up in a health care setting; however, it's my job to speak up, ask the right questions, and get you to tell me what I need to know.

Doctors who communicate well and do their due diligence are known to generate a tremendous rate of positive outcomes for their patients.

EMBRACING A NEW PAIN MANAGEMENT PHILOSOPHY

It's probably apparent by now that my philosophy of chiropractic care is different from that of the medical model's and the one it tries to impose on patients: go to the chiropractor only if you're in pain—otherwise, don't. The result of that, as I've mentioned, is that the pain returns after people stop going to the chiropractor.

Quitting the chiropractor is like saying, "I'm going to leave braces on my teeth for one day and hope everything stays aligned forever once I take them off."

That's crazy.

In those situations, all you and your chiropractor are doing is chasing pain—not correcting any issues or maintaining structural integrity for the future. You're allowing your body to function at less-than-optimal levels.

My philosophy is different. Get rid of your pain, yes—that's what drives patients into my office. But then I educate you on the importance of reducing subluxations and teach you the importance of maintaining good spinal posture and health.

When I put it like that, people understand, but they just have to be educated that this is different from the medical model. This is not a pain-driven modality. This is preventative. This is corrective. This is maintenance.

Just 14 percent of the US population has seen a chiropractor in the last twelve months.[36]

Most people are hesitant to unless they've had a positive experience in the past. That's normal. If you weren't hesitant, I would worry

---

36 GALLUP-PALMER COLLEGE OF CHIROPRACTIC INAUGURAL REPORT: AMERICANS' PERCEPTIONS OF CHIROPRACTIC July 2015.

about you. This is your health, your spine. You should be hesitant about any new procedure or provider.

It's my—and my assistants'—job to put you at ease. We try to do that by giving you the best health care experience you've ever received. That way you learn to trust us, and you learn that we're trained and care about your well-being.

A CUSTOMIZED TREATMENT PLAN DESIGNED SPECIFICALLY FOR YOU

How intensely you need chiropractic adjustments depends on your unique situation. Maybe you'll need it only twice a month. Maybe every day. It just depends.

Recently, a woman brought in her daughter, who had been a dancer for ten years. She showed me a video of her dancing, and I can honestly say she was one of the most beautiful ballet dancers of her age I've ever seen—a gifted girl ... with tremendous back pain. Dancers are hard on their bodies, and the position where they turn out their feet—called the *ballet flagged foot*—may look beautiful, but it causes back and pelvic strain so tremendous that back pain is very common, particularly as these young athletes age.

I did the girl's workup, and as it turned out, her spine and pelvis were out of position.

The dancer's older sister, on the other hand, had a dramatically different problem. She was in pain too, but her problem was a lot easier to correct because she hadn't spent years doing the ballet flagged foot.

That's just an example of how chiropractic isn't a one-size-fits-all treatment—and your adjustments aren't the same every time you come in, either. They change as you progress along the care spectrum.

Each chiropractic visit builds on the one before and gets you ready for the next.

Bodies heal similarly from person to person, but the degree of injury, spinal degeneration, and problems differ from case to case, which is why it's important you find the right chiropractor for you.

SIGNS OF A GOOD DOCTOR

I have several suggestions around this topic based on my experience in the industry. The first and foremost thing is to make sure the chiropractor's beliefs are congruent with yours. Does that mean the chiropractor shouldn't try to educate you about what's best for you? No. However, just like with any other health care provider, they should be on par with your wants, needs, and goals.

Next, make sure they're willing to take the time to educate you, because chiropractic is a process. Your health may never be 100 percent, but as long as you're moving in the right direction toward health and well-being, that's what it's all about.

Beware of providers who don't take time to counsel you on diet or exercise, particularly if they prescribe medication that enables you to continue living a poor lifestyle or recommend that you discontinue physical activity.

Look for providers who take time to go over their report of findings with you, past medical history, and x-rays. It's also a good idea to see an outline of their suggested treatment plan for you in detail.

GOOD LISTENER

I would argue that the attributes you look for in a doctor are the same attributes you look for in a friend or close family member. These providers should be acutely aware of different communication styles and be able to acclimate to these differences, not demand that the patient adhere to their style of communication. A good chiropractor will ask many questions to gain more information or clarify—not to embarrass or attack, but to have a detailed understanding of the patient's health concerns. They seek to be respectful and form partnerships or collaborative relationships with their patients.

Good doctors are not hasty in making judgments. They make evaluations with humility. They are willing to think about something for a while. They don't have to categorize everyone and everything immediately. They consider the angle and point of view from which they are listening. Good chiropractors build a safe environment for you and help you be yourself. They give the patient unthreatened, unhurried space in which to operate while communicating.

Finally, chiropractic doctors who are astute listeners keep eye contact and repeat what they have heard to be sure they have a complete understanding of the patient's situation and have not left any important details out.

PROBLEM SOLVER

A problem-solving professional will redefine the problem. Seasoned chiropractors know that, very often, the initial diagnosis of a patient is often incorrect or incomplete. Problem-solving doctors push further. They go beyond just simply treating pain and find the underlying problem. Why is a patient suffering from arthritis? Why does the patient have sciatica? Why are the discs bulging? Once the chiropractor understands a problem, they then must apply clinical decision-making skills to analyze the patient's case. This analysis should have both short-term (control pain and inflammation) and long-term solutions in mind (fix the problem).

The right chiropractic doctor seeks permanent solutions. The current medical practice approach is very immediate, and concentrated on getting the result right away. Instead, we need to do this right, and consider long-term consequences of these short-term Band-Aid solutions.

The right chiropractor will have a system. The system will approach a patient's case with a structured process that will dramatically increase the chances of successful treatment. It is easy to skip steps and talk about the weather, a current event, or family. A doctor on my team should have the discipline to put aside these distractions and focus on the problem-solving and be sure every step is followed. It should be evident from the initial contact with the support staff that great thought and preparation are dedicated to each patient.

Finally, an excellent chiropractic doctor will consider every patient as if they were their own family member. This is a fundamental way of putting the doctor in the patient's shoes and seeing alternative perspectives to problem solve much more effectively and with empathy. This ability to switch perspectives easily is an attribute of a good chiropractic physician. This characteristic needs to be brought back in a world of impersonal, electronic health care.

EDUCATOR

The chiropractor is constantly learning. They have a passion for teaching others what they have learned, and see difficult cases as opportunities to learn, to grow, to succeed where others have failed. An excellent chiropractor isn't looking for patients to go along with treatment or what is recommended. Instead, we want the patients and their families to understand what we are doing and why we are doing it. The "because I said so" attitude is not acceptable. There must be true understanding by the patient that they concur and are willing to commit to better health. Agreement and concurrence really constitute a very important piece of the permanent solution. This can be done only through patience, education, and the ability to communicate on a level that is well understood by everyone involved. At Advanced Spine & Sports Care, I insist that each staff member master these traits and pledge to be a lifetime student and steward of becoming a good listener, a problem solver, and an educator.

THE REVOLUTIONARY FOUR-PHASE APPROACH TO FUNCTIONAL HEALTH RECOVERY

In my practice, we have four phases a patient can progress to on the care spectrum: relief, correction, strengthening, and supportive. Supportive care is often broken down further depending on the goals and overall health of the patient.

RELIEF CORRECTION STRENGTHENING SUPPORTIVE

RELIEF

The relief phase of care is designed to decrease pain and inflammation. This is generally the most important phase to patients because when they first come in, they're generally in pain. Our goal during this phase is to get you across the pain threshold as quickly as possible and restore as much movement of the spine as we can. By doing that, we're training the body to understand that the area is not an injury site and doesn't require the laying down of inflammation. That will help get rid of the pain.

This is also one of the reasons finding the right chiropractor is important. If you go to the wrong one with an acute injury and they give you a corrective care adjustment, it could likely increase your inflammation and pain. During this phase, patients will generally undergo passive physical therapy and adjustments several times a week as each visit builds on the last. Anti-inflammatory diets are often helpful in this phase as well.

Home care instructions during the first phase of care are fairly simple. Use towels to support the posture we are correcting. Drink half your body weight in ounces of water a day. For example: A two-hundred-pound man should be drinking a hundred ounces of water a day to keep the spine hydrated. Lastly, if the patient experiences any soreness after the adjustments, use ice, not heat. Applying heat may feel good temporarily, but this increases inflammation and often makes the pain worse.

CORRECTION

Next comes the correction phase, where the goals completely change. At this point, the pain should be gone or much improved, meaning many of the pain-relieving treatments performed in the relief phase are no longer necessary.

Often, in this phase, patients will ask me, "Doctor, can't I start strengthening now? I am no longer in pain." The answer is no.

The right phases in the right order will accelerate your journey toward your best health. Shortcuts don't work. Good health and wellness are a process. Trust the process.

During the correction phase, the focus is on correcting problems discovered on the x-ray or problems we already know to exist. For instance, we might correct spinal misalignment, adjust areas that need to be repositioned, or correct pelvic dysfunction. You'll also receive exercises to do at home to maintain that correction. These exercises are designed for neuromuscular reeducation, not strength—to retrain the nervous system to use muscles patients haven't used in years or didn't even know they had. The towel exercise often given in the relief phase, for instance, is now second nature, and I find patients spending more time lying on their backs when in bed.

Often, however, patients don't make it to this phase. They believe that once the pain disappears, they have ten other places they'd rather be, so they disappear too. Then six months, six weeks, or two weeks down the road, they call me because they're in pain again. Why? Because we didn't correct anything. All we did was increase joint function, get rid of inflammation and pain, and just barely take the bone off the nerve. That's it. Once that bone finds the nerve again, we're right back where we started.

That's why this transition from relief to correction is very important. Continuing your care here is the difference between the bone finding the nerve again versus correcting the subluxation. Getting postural muscles identified and explaining their importance around proper spinal alignment plays a critical role in this phase.

STRENGTHENING

The strengthening phase is what most people consider to be physical therapy. However, it's a kind of physical therapy that builds up your entire bodily system—not just the area of concern.

My postdoctoral degree in sports medicine has allowed me to identify the lack of teamwork between the physical therapist and the chiropractic doctor. I understand the importance of muscular imbalance and the role it plays in injury and injury prevention. Everything we do every day, we do the same way. We get into our car the same, work on our computer the same, sit the same. Humans are habitual creatures, but when we predominately use one side of our body, we create an imbalance. Physical therapy can help restore that balance, and in my opinion, that component is as essential as the spinal alignment component. Muscular balance is as important as spinal correction; one without the other is a disservice, particularly when we talk about overall health and wellness. During this phase, we often find that most people working out are using the gym improperly and actually creating more muscular imbalance.

That's why at our clinic we brought those two components—spinal adjustments and physical therapy—together under one roof back in 2002. The physical therapy in my office is prescribed, patient specific, and designed for patients to integrate into their everyday exercise regimens. And if you don't have an exercise regimen, I'll help create one that's laden with the physical therapy I prescribed.

SUPPORTIVE

This phase is a very minimal investment to be sure all the time and effort it takes to get to the "I feel good phase" is not lost. Patients are very happy to reach this phase. At my office, we transition people from patients to practice members. This is a clear distinction. When patients become practice members, we are creating lasting habits in diet, exercise, and overall health and wellness. Adjustments occur much less frequently and we concentrate on strengthening the nervous system. This shift to preventative mindsets increases sports performance and decreases the incidence of injury. Now, I would be remiss if I didn't mention that not everyone sees the value of this phase and falls out of care. Unfortunately, this then leads to practice members becoming patients again and having to repeat some if not all of these phases again. This is obviously not ideal and why we really focus on education and the importance of the wellness phase.

For the majority of my patients, this four-phase approach works exceptionally well. However, for some who have a bulge or herniated disc that doesn't respond to traditional chiropractic care, a more intensive treatment is needed: spinal decompression.

CHAPTER TAKEAWAYS:

- Chiropractic care is often made to fit into a medical paradigm, so it is frequently centered around pain, but is so much more than that.

- Our revolutionary four-phase approach to functional health recovery gets you out of pain, corrects the problem, and strengthens your body around proper alignment.

- Spinal misalignment is no more important than the muscular imbalance and weakness that perpetuate these alignment problems.

Chapter 6

SPINAL DECOMPRESSION: IS IT RIGHT FOR YOU?

For most people, back pain is just an annoyance we shouldn't have to live with, but we do. For one patient, Matt, it was more than that: back pain was ruining his career. A jiujitsu competitor who'd won multiple titles, Matt had hurt his back and could no longer walk, never mind train or compete.

He worked with his physician to seek out cures, and eventually, the physician recommended he have surgery because of the severe bulge—4.5 millimeters, to be exact—in his L5 disc. After that consult, however, Matt was skeptical about surgery as the best route. He'd researched the statistics—less than half of fusion surgeries succeed in returning the patient to their preinjury condition. He also knew that once the procedure was performed, there was no going back, so he paid me a visit to see if he had other options.

After some preliminary examinations, I discovered his bulge was so severe that it was narrowing the disc spaces within his spine, putting pressure on the nerves traveling through it. His problem was bad—too bad, in fact, for regular alignments to be effective.

After the consultation, exam, imaging, and education, we decided that nonsurgical spinal decompression was his best and least risky treatment option. Spinal decompression is reserved for extremely difficult cases and is the only nonsurgical treatment that can sufficiently relieve pressure on the disc, allowing the body to heal itself naturally. It's designed for patients who have herniated discs, bulging discs, or degenerative disc disease that impinge on nerves, causing pain. There's also little to no risk of the injury getting worse from the treatment, which is a major bonus.

WHAT DECOMPRESSION IS ALL ABOUT

Decompression is a buzzword that's used a lot these days, but in the chiropractic world, it refers to a particular machine that applies angular force on the spine so that various discs can be treated differently. Computer technology controls not only the pressure on the spine, but the angle at which this pressure is applied. It occurs slowly and in phases, effectively preventing the body from responding as it naturally would, which is by contracting the muscles.

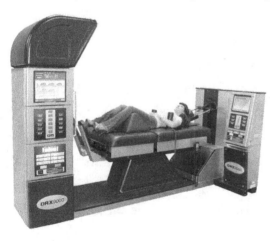

Put simply, decompression allows a very slight separation so that the spine can reabsorb disc material into normal confines, where it belongs. For bulging discs (which is something your MRI or CT scan may reveal), studies show that spinal decompression can lower the pressure inside the disc.[37]

Patients who consider this therapy have usually tried just about everything, but their cases are so severe that this treatment is their best hope.

The principle behind the therapy is simple:

- The disc is a cushion-like material that sits between the bones of the spine, keeping them from rubbing together and giving you the flexibility to safely move your back. When discs are injured or degenerate, lingering pain and impaired movement usually occur.

- Back pain can be caused by nerve pressure created from bulged or herniated spinal disc tissue.

- Nonsurgical decompression therapy is administered using a sophisticated FDA-cleared machine that gently stretches the spine and decompresses discs while causing little to no discomfort.

- In addition to taking pressure off the discs, the slow, controlled stretching creates a vacuum that naturally sucks displaced, bulging disc material back toward the center of the discs and away from your nerves.

- Once the pressure on the nerves is released, they can begin to heal. (Much like what happens when you take pressure off a broken foot.)

---

37 Christian C. Apfel et al., "Restoration of disk height through non-surgical spinal decompression is associated with decreased discogenic low back pain: a retrospective cohort study," *BMC Musculoskeletal Disorders* 11 (2010): 155. https://doi.org/10.1186/1471-2474-11-155.

Because each patient responds differently, the results from decompression can vary from patient to patient. For instance, many patients feel a difference within two to three treatments; others feel them immediately.

The theory behind spinal decompression stems from traction or inversion therapy, various forms of treatment that have been around for more than a thousand years. However, spinal decompression is different from traction and has improved on that concept—decompression therapy decompresses specific discs, while traction pulls each disc the same amount, whether it needs it or not.

Hanging upside down is a commonly used method to put the spine into axial traction. In this method, we leverage gravity to remove force and pressure from the spine rather than put stress on it, which is what happens when we stand upright.

The idea of traction is geared in the right direction, except its 180-degree pull means the L1 disc space is treated the same way as the L5 disc space.

If you look at the spine from the side, you'll notice it's curved. Here's why: The spine sits on the bone called the *sacrum*. The sacrum is a large wedge-shaped vertebra at the bottom (inferior end) of the spine that lies between the fifth disc of the lumbar spine (L5) and the coccyx (tailbone). It forms the solid base of the spinal column where it intersects with the hip bones to form the pelvis. The sacrum is a strong bone that supports the weight of the upper body as it's spread across the pelvis and into the legs. The L5 disc and vertebrae are not square to the sacrum; it's angled downward depending on how steep the patient's sacrum is from birth. The L4 is also angular, as are the L3 and L2, which is what produces what we call the *lordotic curve*, or the low back curve.

True decompression takes those curves and angles into account; axial traction does not.

Several clinical studies have shown traction to be an ineffective form of back and neck pain relief, where the pain relief is inconsistent and short lived.[38] The reason for that is pretty simple: when the spine is pulled, our bodies respond by contracting or squeezing the muscles around it. Rather than achieving the desired effect of taking pressure off the spine, traction actually increases the pressure on it, thereby also increasing pressure in the discs. This means that discs aren't able to rehydrate and heal, which are key factors that ultimately yield pain relief.

Spinal decompression machines, on the other hand, sense your muscles' resistance to the pulling forces and cycle the pull so that your body does not resist the tension, making it much more effective.

The machine also is gentle in its stretching of the back, so pain and discomfort are unlikely—in fact, many of my patients fall asleep during treatment.

I'm one of only three chiropractors in Illinois who offers spinal decompression utilizing the DRX9000, and the only one in Chicago. Why is that so if decompression is truly as effective as experts say? Mainly it has to do with the cost of the equipment and the lack of

---

38   For some examples, see M. Hiranandani, "Non-surgical spinal decompression—treatment of low back pain by spinal decompression and spinal exercises." Paper presented at the forty-fifth annual India Association of Physiotherapy Conference, February 1–4, 2007; N. Oi et al., "Effects of spinal decompression (DRX9000) for lumbar disc herniation," *Journal of Saitama Kenou Rehabilitation* 6 (November 1, 2006); J. Leslie, "Prospective evaluation of the efficacy of spinal decompression via the DRX9000 for chronic low back pain," *Journal of Medicine* (September 2008); A. Macario, "Systematic literature review of spinal decompression via motorized traction for chronic discogenic low back pain," *Pain Practice* 6, no. 3 (2006): 171–178.

WHO IT'S RIGHT FOR

	Pros	Cons
Nonsurgical spinal decompression:	• Very high success rate—Better than seven out of ten cases • Painless—Many patients fall asleep during treatment Drug free • Very safe—Virtually impossible to end up worse than where you started • Costs a tenth of the amount of most surgeries • Can help with many conditions that other treatments like surgery, chiropractic, and physical therapy cannot	• A very small percentage of patients see no difference after treatment
Surgery:	• Some patients experience permanent pain relief	• Risk—A last resort that carries the risk of making your symptoms worse postprocedure • Low success rate—Many procedures have less than a 50 percent success rate • Painful and long recovery time • Very expensive
Pain pills:	• Immediate pain relief	• Not a lasting solution—Similar to taking a painkiller to deal with a toothache caused by a cavity—No amount of pills will fix the cause of your pain • Without the pain, you are more likely to reinjure yourself • 16,500 people die and 103,000 people are hospitalized each year because of NSAID-related problems [39]
Nerve blocks/spinal injections:	• Immediate pain relief	• Not a lasting solution—Similar to taking a painkiller to deal with a toothache caused by a cavity. No amount of pills will fix the cause of pain • Without the pain, you're more likely to reinjure yourself • Very expensive
Bed rest:	• Sometimes works	• Puts your life on hold, possibly for months • Can make your condition worse, as muscles become weaker from lack of use • Weak muscles make you more likely to reinjure yourself

Physical therapy:	• Can provide permanent pain relief • Low risk	• Low success rate with chronic and lingering conditions • Treatment can take months, if not years
Traction:	• Some patients experience relief	• Rarely effective—The body naturally resists spinal pull, so it tenses up the muscles. Because it is impossible to stop using our spine, there will always be pressure on an injury, never allowing it to heal • In some cases, the battle between the body and the traction pull can make conditions worse
Doing nothing or "waiting it out":	• Works for the mildest conditions	• Left untreated, most patients get worse. It's not possible to stop using the back or neck and thus relieve pressure on the injury, which is necessary for healing to occur. • A recipe for disaster in most cases • Many people who choose this option end up as candidates for back surgery

insurance reimbursement. I bought the DRX9000 fifteen years ago when it cost $125,000; I'm not sure what the cost is now, but that's a steep investment for a treatment option that isn't frequently used. However, that purchase was one of the best decisions I've made in my professional career.

When I started offering this treatment in 2003, it was still new. Because I got in early, I've been involved in many of the original case studies and research on the machine, including national conference calls with doctors to discuss treatment protocols, best practices, and what's worked best for the toughest cases. I've discovered that, by far, decompression is the best option for treating bulges or herniations that don't respond to other conservative treatments.

Whether it's a thirteen-millimeter bulge or two-millimeter bulge, if I can change that bulge by a millimeter, it can make all the difference in the world in eliminating the patient's symptoms.

To make spinal decompression as effective as possible, the first step is making sure the diagnosis is correct. That means making sure the primary cause of the pain is the bulge and/or herniated disc. Many patients come in and say they have a bulging disc, but in actuality, the bulging disc isn't what is causing their pain. It can certainly be a complicating factor, but it isn't the primary cause of the discomfort. For example, a patient may come in and say, "I've got pain that goes down my right leg, and I've got pain in my lower back." Their MRI will show a left-sided bulge. A bulge to the left nerves is not going to cause radiating pain in the right side of the body, so we need to figure out exactly what's going on and make sure we're taking care of the right problem. So the first step is making sure the diagnosis is accurate and congruent with the patient's symptoms. I do that by examining their MRI and actively listening.

Some patients tell me they had spinal decompression at another office and it really helped them. I'll say, "Okay. Show me your MRI."

"I never had an MRI," they'll reply.

This stumps me. Without an MRI, how could the doctor have even known what they were treating? How could they have known which discs to target? Consulting the MRI, and educating the patient about what it says, is a vital part of the process.

There is a hierarchy of candidacy for spinal decompression, meaning that there are people who are excellent candidates, good candidates, fair candidates, or not candidates at all. It's not a one-size-fits-all treatment. In my office, I use spinal decompression only on those who are good or excellent candidates.

One significant variable that dictates treatment is the number of segments involved. The best candidates will have just one bulge or herniation. However, usually, if a patient has an L5 bulge or herniation, they may also have an L4, L3, or L2 bulge/herniation—

particularly if they've been dealing with this problem for a year or more. If the patient has two levels of involvement—for example, two bulges—they automatically go from an excellent candidate to, at best, a good candidate. When we get into the actual examination and consultation is when I learn more about whether or not they'll be a candidate at all.

People who have had hardware installed in their back, severe osteoporosis, or any type of active fracture or infection are not candidates for spinal decompression.

HOW THE TREATMENT AND PROCESS WORK

The treatment plan varies by patient and individual conditions, and creating it is a bit of an art. The amount of pressure used and the length of time I treat the patient are based on their presentation and problem. Generally, treatments last thirty to forty-five minutes each and occur three to five times a week for four to six weeks.

During treatment, the patient lies face up, knees bent, hands relaxed, and with support rests underneath their shoulders.

The DRX9000 produces a computer-generated sine wave of pressure that is repetitively applied and released so as not to make the patient feel there's a large amount of weight applied all at once. This technique is what guards against muscle contraction. Nine times out of ten, patients can't even tell where or how much pressure is being applied. Most claim they feel no pressure at all, and that's exactly what we want.

For patients experiencing significant amounts of pain, the only time they feel relief is when they're lying on that table during treatment.

Once decompression is complete, we administer ice and inter-ferential current just in case muscle spasms occur—which is rare but not unheard of.

To continue to protect and relax the muscles, thereby increas-ing the effectiveness of the treatment, the patient will then wear a decompression belt during waking hours.

A good spinal decompression treatment plan will teach the body that the bulge or herniation isn't an injury site anymore. The reason surgeries fail so regularly is that treating the bulge doesn't do anything. It's not the actual bulge that puts pressure on the nerve. Rather the bulge creates an injury site that then lays down inflamma-tion, which is what is really responsible for the pressure on the nerve.

Spinal decompression can solve that problem without surgery.

The good news is, once you've completed treatment, you're done. Physical therapy is often prescribed to help strengthen the area once decompression is complete. There has not been any research suggest-ing continued sessions have any long-term benefit. Matt, from the beginning of this chapter, had terrific results from spinal decompres-sion. Soon after treatment, he was back to competing on the mat, and to this day he still hasn't had any problems. Not only did we alleviate the herniation, but we also taught his body that his lower back wasn't an injury site. Every thirty days or so, Matt comes back in for a chiropractic adjustment, and around his treatments, he's out there winning national and international titles. Matt understands the importance of the wellness phase and how it plays a vital role in his career.

If you're a good or an excellent candidate for spinal decompres-sion, I'm convinced my treatment approach will have you doing the things you love again. For some people that means competitive sports; for others, it means being able to pick up their grandchildren again.

CHAPTER TAKEAWAYS:

- For the most severe cases of disc bulges or herniations, spinal decompression offers the best option for treatment.

- Spinal decompression is a noninvasive, pain-free stretching of individual spinal bones that allows the disc material to return to its natural position.

39   Centers for Disease Control and Prevention. Vital signs: Overdoses of prescription opioid pain relievers and other drugs among women— United States, 1999–2010. Morbidity and Mortality Weekly Report 62, no. 26 (2013): 537–542.

CONCLUSION

My father, who once called chiropractors "glorified massage thera-pists," recently pointed out to me that *Family Practice Journal* now recommends patients seek chiropractic care for musculoskeletal low back pain before turning to traditional medical care. He has visited a chiropractor himself. Many hospitals and group practices are incor-porating physical medicine and rehabilitation services such as chiro-practic into their networks.

His opinion has certainly changed over the years.

Hospitals, in general, are slowly starting to embrace chiroprac-tic, primarily because they have to; change is coming, and they can either capitalize off it or be left behind by competitors who do.

With this change is coming a gradual-but-growing respect for what chiropractors do.

People my age and younger (let's say midforties and younger) are more likely to understand that traditional treatments for certain medical conditions aren't appropriate. It used to be that the doctor was considered all knowing and the doctor's advice would be heeded without question; if my grandmother's medical doctor had told her that the way to treat her ailment was to cut off her head, she'd have done it. I remember her telling me, "If the doctor says to do something, then that's what needs to be done."

Nowadays it's different. Whether because of increased awareness or increased cost responsibility, people are asking more questions, becoming more proactive in their own health care, and becoming more educated consumers. As a result, they see the shortcomings in the current medical model and the value of alternative therapies—and they're more likely to get what chiropractic can do for them.

They're also starting to understand that, when comparing cost and value of chiropractic versus medical care, chiropractic wins every time. The possibility of medication addiction isn't worth it. The cost-benefit of surgery, not to mention the limited likelihood of success, risks, and downtime, isn't worth it.

However, we still have a long way to go before chiropractic is used as it should be—as a complementary practice in your regular health care regimen, right alongside your primary care physician and dentist.

Chiropractic is about much more than aligning the spine so that it functions properly. It's also a lifestyle change. It's a return to the previous model where doctors counsel patients about lifestyle and exercise. Chiropractors counsel patients about things they can do to make a big difference in their lives—not just relevant to their longevity but also to the quality of their lives.

Today's physicians' offices, with their get-them-in-get-them-out environments, don't have the time or see the need to get back to basic health care. We fill that gap. By doing so, we can help solve the problems of the health care crisis—such as opioid addiction, needless and ineffective surgeries, and high costs that this country is experiencing today. The chiropractic philosophy is to try natural treatments first and medicine last.

Chiropractic can't fix everything. However, if your problem is neck, shoulder, back, hip, or leg related, or has to do with any of the other issues I talked about in chapter 3, you owe it to yourself to explore a natural fix before seeking more extreme options.

If your back pain, or neck pain, is caused by something other than a pinched or irritated nerve—say, for example, kidney disease or a liver problem—we're trained to identify that and send you to the proper specialist. However, you can't get surgery first and then try chiropractic to fix the problem if the surgery proves unsuccessful.

If you've made it this far, then I've said something that's resonated with you. I may have upset you a little—and I hope I did. I hope I made you angry. I hope I made you question what you're doing with your medical care, so in the end, you can make a more informed decision for your body.

ABOUT MY CHIROPRACTIC PRACTICE

I have a certified chiropractic sports physician distinction above and beyond my chiropractic degree, so I've learned everything from sideline treatment to emergency medical care, including advanced cardiac life support and much more. This means I look at things a little differently than most chiropractors.

My practice is a journey, not a destination. I am here to serve my patients and my community. It's always been my job to listen, learn, and evolve as a practitioner and as the owner of a practice. I believe my ability to change, keep abreast of the latest research, and improve treatment standards based on that research are the factors that have helped contribute to my success.

When I became a chiropractor, I never imagined just how powerful, how life altering, what I do would become. However, every so often, I'm reminded of it. A few months ago, for instance, I got an email from a girl who was a patient of mine. As we had worked through the four components of treatment, we discovered that the emotional aspect of her pain was a large factor for her, to the point that she was hospitalized a few times for psych evaluation.

The email she sent me said, "I just want you to know, Dr. Ingham, that you saved my life. The time that you took with me, the help that you gave me to not only relieve my pain but also to educate me on the wrong path I was going down, saved my life."

It is those kinds of comments that make me stop and think, "Whoever would have thought that a lowly chiropractor from Detroit, Michigan, would get an email like that?"

It's pretty cool. The other correspondences I receive are not all quite that dramatic, but I get several a month telling me what a difference I've made in someone's life.

Honestly, I never expected that chiropractic would afford me so many great things. My initial thought process was always along the lines of, "We're back doctors. We're pain doctors." However, for the people who are on the receiving end of it, it's much more than that—so much beyond the physical component—as I've discussed throughout this book.

FINAL THOUGHTS

As I wrap up, I'd like to leave you with this thought: living a long life isn't enough. What good is it to be eighty-three years old if you can't get out of your wheelchair, or bathe yourself? If you can't play with your grandchildren, or travel to new places?

During my lectures, I often ask people in the audience how many of them want to live until they're eighty-three. Most people raise their hands—but not all. I pick on those who don't raise their hands, asking, "Why is it that you don't want to live to be eighty-three?" The response is almost always some version of, "If it means I'll feel proportionally worse than I do today, I don't want to get that old."

No matter how many times I hear it (and it's often), it's still a horrible response—I can't believe that someone would rather be dead than alive because they are afraid of feeling physically worse than they do now. That means they are potentially willing to give up years of their life—missed birthdays, weddings, graduations, sunsets, laughs, special moments—all to avoid feeling physical pain.

But it doesn't have to be that way. It starts by taking action now, so you don't feel bad at eighty-three, or even today, for that matter. A body in motion stays in motion, and just the opposite is true as well. Inaction triggers a vicious cycle. Many patients say the reason they're not active is because something hurts—their back, their knees, their hips. In turn, they give up exercise. Then their back or hips hurt more because they're not exercising. Throughout this cycle, the ability to move freely slows down and prevents them from living their lives to the fullest.

Chiropractic is the answer. It will help get your body back in motion, so you can continue doing what you love to do. I hope reading this book has caused you to question your medical care up to this point and encouraged you to think about how you approach your health. I even hope that reading this has made you mad at times. While it isn't, and never is, my intention to disregard any specialty or modality, it is imperative for patients to know that there are other options available that don't involve going under the knife or taking a myriad of pills. If I've shared something that struck you and you want to learn more, contact my staff or me personally. Maybe you know a friend or family member who needs help. Or, if you're the one in pain, what are you waiting for? Fix the reason for the pain. Now.

There is hope for healing those aches and pains and leading a pain-free life. I know it because I live one, and such insight has carried over to my philosophy of practice and has set my high standards for care. Pain isn't a natural, inevitable result of aging. We can fix it together, or—best of all—prevent it from happening in the first place.

Go on … book the plane tickets with your wife. Say yes to throwing a baseball around with your grandson or taking an afternoon hiking with your friends.

Call our office now—we're ready to help you get back to living. Are you?

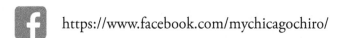 https://www.facebook.com/mychicagochiro/

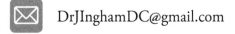 DrJInghamDC@gmail.com

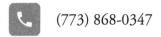 (773) 868-0347

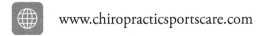 www.chiropracticsportscare.com